Living On
the Margins

Living On the Margins

Women Writers on Breast Cancer

EDITED, WITH AN INTRODUCTION BY HILDA RAZ

A Karen *and* Michael Braziller Book

PERSEA BOOKS / NEW YORK

Acknowledgments

This book was helped by many people. Robin Becker, Charlotte Sheedy, and Karen Braziller brought it to print. Marilyn Hacker was a steady advance woman as she has been for so many literary projects. Maxine Kumin solicited essays. Aaron Link saw me through the introduction. Ladette Randolph, managing editor of *Prairie Schooner,* gave at the office during the summer of final manuscript preparation. John Link, Maria Schoenhammer, and Constance Merritt were available as they were needed. The writers of this book who entertained my ideas, made art from illness, jokes from suffering, life from death—to them everything.

Persea Books, Inc.
171 Madison Avenue
New York, New York 10016

Library of Congress Cataloging-in-Publication Data

Living on the margins : women writers on breast cancer / edited, with an
    introduction by Hilda Raz.
            p.   cm.
    "A Karen and Michael Braziller Book."
    ISBN 0-89255-244-1 (hbk. : alk. paper)
    1. Breast—Cancer.   2. Breast—Cancer Poetry.   I. Raz. Hilda.
    II. Title: Women writers on breast cancer.
    RC280.B8L54   1999
    362. 1'9699449—dc21   99-32917
                                                      CIP

Printed and bound by R. R. Donnelly & Company
Text designed by Rita Lascaro
FIRST EDITION

Contents

Introduction: Writing On the Margins *by Hilda Raz* vii

Cancer Says *by Pamela Post* 3

Off *by Maxine Kumin* 18

A Design Upon Us *by Judith Hall* 27

St. Peregrinus' Cancer (poem) *by Judith Hall* 37

"C"-ing in Colors *by Safiya Henderson-Holmes* 40

The Good Mother *by Annette Williams Jaffee* 46

White Glasses *by Eve Kosofsky Sedgwick* 57

Lateral Time *by Carole Simmons Oles* 76

Interview with Susan Love, M.D. *by Carole Simmons Oles* 98

Bone Scan (poem) *by Amy Ling* 112

The Alien Within *by Amy Ling* 114

Getting Well (poem) *by Hilda Raz* 134

Flowers, Bones *by Claudia MonPere McIsaac* 136

"No communion with despair": Kay Boyle on Cancer
by Sandra Spanier 156

Poems *by Lucille Clifton* 170

Scenes from a Mastectomy *by Alicia Ostriker* 175

Journal Entries *by Marilyn Hacker* 201

The Other Redhead and Me *by Mimi Schwartz* 242

Poems *by Carol Dine* 250

From the Front Line *by Carol Dine* 254

The Scan Chronicles *by Janet Sternburg* 260

Telling *by Elaine Greene* 274

Biographical Notes on the Authors 282

Introduction: Writing On *the* Margins

I love a broad margin to my life.
—Henry David Thoreau

IT'S SUMMER. IN THE GARDEN TWO WOMEN ARE
cutting up fruit for lunch. One takes a golden peach, twists free the
pit. She hands half to her friend, points to a spot of mold attached
to the stem. "No problem," the other grins, twirling her knife. She
hands back the half. "Clean margins," she whispers. They both
laugh. Clean margins around a compromised site may indicate
successful treatment for cancer. The women use medical language
for their own delight. Their laughter spreads through this book.

Women in gardens has been a popular subject for art, a double
image of nature tamed by culture. But the women in this garden
might be seen as nature run riot. Each has given up a breast to
treatment for cancer. Both understand their loss is hidden. Each
knows this amputation is different from others, the breast an erotic,
sexual, and maternal emblem in a culture that reveres breasts if not
women. They live on the margins of communities where anecdotes
of suffering about breast cancer are told by healthy friends on the
leveraged margins of chance and luck. Each has searched the work
of women writers for records of direct experience. Neither can find
them. The absence is odd. Why is an experience so common and
transformative so notably absent in contemporary literature? A
margin of missing literature surrounds breast cancer. One example
might stand for others. Pioneer environmentalist Rachel Carson
had breast cancer and chose not to mention it in her best-selling
Silent Spring (1962), although she made clear the connection
between DDT, illness, and death. Her reticence seems to define a

long tradition of silence. If silence = death, as we have learned from AIDS activists, where are the artists living with breast cancer? What margins of silence confine them? Where is their work? Why should we all care?

One of the functions of culture, the work of the human mind, is to explain experience and the world we inhabit. An unexpected life-changing event forces us to the limits of culture. There are places where the rational mind is helpless. Cancer is certainly one of them; in fact it may be the archetype of this kind of incomprehensible ordeal. In traditional epistemologies in which the healthy body is understood as orderly, cancer is defined as chaos, nature run riot, the physical antithesis of culture. "Body my house/my horse my hound," wrote poet May Swenson, "what will I do/when you are fallen?" Swenson articulates a traditional sense of the body as mind's shelter and companion; a contemporary book about women's health pushes the notion, equates body and mind in its title *Our Bodies, Ourselves.* A woman *is* her body. Cancer that threatens the breast, the marker of gender and the maternal, the female erotic and aesthetic, may also threaten traditional definitions of identity, as many men with breast cancer may attest. Any damage to the breast provides a paradigm of extreme experience, one that pushes against the boundaries of the rational mind and challenges the impulses that lead the mind to construct and accept culture.

Artists are both builders and consumers of culture. They work with expectations that define what they write, how they write, and what their readers should be encouraged to consider. So artists, who have been called iconoclasts, destroyers of icons, questioners of cultures and their institutions, often begin by making new images of a bounded world their culture tells them to see. But artists also are trained to resist and transgress the margins of cultural expectations. Susan Sontag provides one example in her book *Illness as Metaphor,* in which she notes the judgment of moral depravity that cancer carries in twentieth-century America—like a "bad" gene on DNA, like tuberculosis in European culture in the nineteenth century. Perhaps artists with breast cancer have two choices: to confine their work to familiar boundaries of "moral failure"—guilt, suffering, and atonement—or to confront the failure of the rational mind to make working explanations for their experience by retreating and falling silent, by refusing to fill the page.

As an editor and writer, I wanted to find a third choice: writing on the margins that isolate breast cancer patients. I wanted to discover ways writers accept the risk cancer brings and use it in their work. I wanted artists to engage the failure of available cancer paradigms by disassembling them and claiming an extended field. It seemed to me that writers could articulate both the substance of their experience and also a reparative response to inadequate stories about the body, illness in general, cancer, and especially breast cancer. By making art that repairs and expands conventional images of their bodies and their lives, artists might repair the world that encloses and threatens to bankrupt patient and their families and friends.

The makers of this book are artists by profession. I invited them to make public their work—essays, shaped journals, poems, and scholarly articles—about what was so notably absent. They delivered for the most part work remarkably devoid of paranoid readings of their experience. In a society that takes apart women for erotic or commercial reasons, these writers confronted treatment for breast cancer that is, in the famous phrase of breast cancer surgeon Dr. Susan Love, "slash, poison, and burn. " They encountered, witnessed, and documented traditional and alternative treatments by medical practitioners in the nineteenth century as well as the twentieth. They recovered letters and historical documents by women writers and told family stories. They worked, in the words of poet Judith Hall, from "compulsion and utility." And they delivered texts in the spirit of Eve Kosofsky Sedgwick, who wrote in her watershed essay, "White Glasses," "in many ways it is full of stimulation and interest, even, to be ill and writing." Audre Lorde in 1980 in *The Cancer Journals* said, "I would never have chosen this path, but I am very glad to be who I am, here." These writers present themselves and their progenitors not as heroic but efficient. They are efficient in their use of crisis to carry on their lives as writers. They use easily what comes to hand, to smash and rebuild. Making art is their profession, and in this collection their material is cancer. The joy with which they do their chosen work, even at the apparent limits of human endurance, is everywhere present.

When poet Gertrude Stein wrote, "A rose is a rose is a rose," she might have been saying a rose is a flower, not a woman. Her distrust of metaphor is famous. Writers perpetuate and deconstruct cultures by analyzing, rearranging, and synthesizing experience and expectations. They give faces and names to stories, complicated amalgams of political and personal experience. They often use metaphor to help us understand difference, lives unlike our own, powerful and dangerous forces, the extremes of human interaction with each other and our environment. Metaphor can help us to understand experiences alien and unfamiliar in our lives. But metaphor also can be used to simplify complex ideas or express and perpetuate common assumptions. It can erase gradations of difference by addressing opposites: good and evil, for example. Health and illness. Conservation and profit. Culture and nature. Risk and reward. Men and women. Disclosure and decorum. Black and white. We all know metaphors that express cancer as the devil, the betrayer. Crisis doesn't care. In crisis our familiar limits, containments, margins are broken, proved useless. The writers of this book have chosen to repair their lives after the experience of breast cancer in ways important for everyone. We all live inside the common assumptions of our cultures. We need to know this shelter is illusory before we can take the tools of repair into our own hands.

Certainly no writer in this book expected cancer in her life. Each one responds differently. But each engages through her work the fracture of her expectations. It's important to look at this work because each writer has traveled beyond the margins of the known world, beyond the limits of culture, beyond the boundaries of what can be explained by the rational world, a place we all must go, writer or not. Each brings back to us news that stays news, Ezra Pound's definition of art.

What exactly is the job of the writer? Linda McCarriston suggests in her essay "Class Unconsciousness and an American Writer" that

[t]he job of the writer is ... to present one world to another world, to present one life to another life, a hidden life to one who would, by and large, prefer not to know it. That which is hidden is hidden for a reason. To reveal it is to make someone uncomfortable—or responsible, let's say. To reveal what has been hidden entails, on the part of the writer, a *de facto* awareness of the gap between these two [reader and writer], as well as an awareness of the resistance of "the reader" to know, truly, the life heretofore hidden. Not knowing, ignoring, is bliss, insofar as bliss is an equilibrium in which one finds oneself safe and comfortable. Horace's injunction that art must both teach and delight then becomes the task of the writer and the key to revealing what has been hidden, seducing the reluctant knower with the pleasure, the intellectual thrill, the "terrible beauty" of the unwanted lesson: into knowing.

It's no accident that the media sends experienced writers into situations of danger to witness and report, describe life in its extremities to audiences safely at home. Language is a powerful tool for empathy. It opens the borders between us, helps us understand difference. The audience for memoir and reportage at the millennium is great. These essays are both. If readers have become accustomed to a posture of paranoia, discovering in every book and film evidence of cultural bad news, perhaps the essays in this book demonstrate the pleasures of a reparative response. Here's joy in the making, joy in the narrative, joy in the deciphering, joy in the language, the pun, the comparison: critic, poet, and essayist Alicia Ostriker's "Scenes from a Mastectomy" is not Ingmar Bergman's "Scenes from a Marriage" but owns a seriousness of intent and a playfulness of contrast. And it seems to me that the joy in making these essays and poems affects even their assigned sad subjects, their expression of grief over the body's mechanisms gone wrong, the predation of our environment. This work also presents new paradigms and narratives as their makers begin to construct ways to analyze and represent lives altered by cancer.

This collection of essays offers no conclusions, no unified perspective. The requirements for inclusion were two overlapping sets of experience. The first one is a choice, to wish to know ourselves as writers. The second no one would choose. We each one have felt terror and despair about breast cancer. Ostriker articulates it: "Between the forces arrayed against us within our own cells, and the forces of human nature acted out on the scale of human history, each of us is almost entirely helpless." And then she adds, "although we can perhaps do little to heal either the world or ourselves, we can do *something*. Something is not the same as nothing." The pieces range from Safiya Henderson-Holmes's vision of racial difference "in a stark, white hospital, my black female body between its sheets, sutured and gauzed, pierced with tubing...I am another 'other'..." through Carole Simmons Oles's account of her refusal to be colonized by a medical system that both botched and provided care, to her interview with breast cancer surgeon, activist, and writer Dr. Susan Love, under whose aegis the boundaries of care are rearranged, the margins of acceptable treatment revised. Pulitzer Prize-winner Maxine Kumin responds to mastectomy by refusing to wear the prosthesis her insurance company provides and tucks an old shoulder pad into her bathing suit. Prize-winning poet, translator, and critic Marilyn Hacker offers selected journals of her illness and surgery, insight and information about her time as editor of *Kenyon Review* during months of treatment and travel between her homes in New York City, Ohio, and Paris. When she fusses, "much easier to approach this disease as if it were my recovery from a traumatic motorcycle crackup" she speaks to gendered notions of suffering. Judith Hall recalls nineteenth-century novelist Fanny Burney's surgery without anesthesia, and scholar Sandra Spanier edits unpublished letters of the Lost

Generation writer, Kay Boyle. Spanier shows the graphic intersection of the political and personal in Boyle's life, in prison in 1968 as a Vietnam War protester when she discovered the lump in her breast. "...I went to the lock-up shower, where plywood nailed across the window took the place of sawed-through bars and broken glass. It was then, as I soaped myself up and down and back and forth under the strong, warm needles of water, that I felt the lump for the first time. It was very small. It was really nothing. When I dried myself, it was still there. By six-thirty in the morning, when the cart creaked up the hall with breakfast for one and all, it had not gone away."

We learn from Judith Hall that the name of the patron saint of cancer, Peregrinus, means "'crossing the field'; going away, one-legged," and we meet, in Annette Williams Jaffee's brilliant account of genetic risk, in her surgeon's office, Saint Agatha, the patron saint of breast diseases, "her naked outstretched arms offering her own breasts like bonbons on a silver platter." Pioneer scholar of Asian American literature and poet Amy Ling recalls her life as student and professor, perceived by colleagues as alien within a hostile, sexist, and racist American university system, "labeled a cancer, harboring cancer, fighting to eliminate cancer." Anthologist Janet Sternburg chronicles risk and friendship over a decade of repeated medical scans and examinations. The roles and relationships of mother and daughter form a matrix for Claudia MonPere McIsaac and Annette Williams Jaffee. Lucille Clifton asks, "what is the splendor of one breast/on one woman?"

Audre Lorde, our most powerful contemporary progenitor, contextualized her illness in a catalogue of identities—black, lesbian, mother, writer, activist. She never believed her cancer was natural in a world of cultural—political, social, and environmental—atrocities. Nor did she, nor can any of the writers in this book provide a simple discourse of breast cancer, nor a single politics or aesthetic. Only language itself can remake the margins, revise the text, express the ratio of risk to reward, posit cultural change. For breast cancer patients, a clean margin around a cancerous site suggests containment, possible recovery. The alternative, dirty margins, suggests cancer uncontained, more surgery, chemotherapy, and/or radiation. We all hope for clean margins in the body. None of us respects them on the page. We accept risk as writers who live on the margins, placing our trust in future readers of our work. Whatever we may wish, every one of us here in fact lives forever on the margins.

Kay Boyle suggested that the human tragedy of individual isolation ironically might be overturned by illness or imprisonment. I believe that language can save us from isolation. As a writer, teacher, and editor of the literary journal *Prairie Schooner,* I've read many accounts of crisis, many more than any journal can publish. Most demonstrate the ways art intersects with life and document the place of public policy—poverty, racism, pollution, chemical overflow, war—in private lives. As Ostriker writes in reference to the Gulf War, "I must cling to accuracy in language, in this age of euphemistic rot when...we live in a verbal drizzle of acceptable losses, collateral damage, deterrent, non-combatant....Surgical strike....It is a tiny war, a speck of a war. Like the insignificant speck of cancer in my breast a few months ago."

I too had a breast cancer diagnosis, mine made in 1990, nine months after major surgery, before my recovery was complete. Treatment included more surgery, mastectomy. In 1990 the figures that represented quantifiable data told me that 1 in 10 women during the course of her lifetime will have breast cancer. Now the figure is 1 in 8. I seem to bear witness: the most recent contributor to *Living On the Margins* is Carole Simmons Oles, close friend and collaborator on several literary projects. This book takes its place in our growing bibliography. I would have preferred not. In 1990, I had daily news of new colleagues in treatment. Now, in America, a woman dies of breast cancer every twelve minutes, around the clock. Nor is the epidemic confined to U.S. borders, or to women. According to Cathy Read's introduction to *Cancer Through the Eyes of Ten Women* (London:

Pandora Press, 1997), "Breast cancer is the most common cancer among women in the world; it killed 560,000 women in 1980 and is predicted to claim the lives of one million women annually by the year 2000." In the United States, male breast cancer accounts for one of every hundred cases and accounts for about .2 percent of all malignancies in men. According to the National Cancer Institute's SEER program, breast cancer affects fourteen black men and eight white men in every million. Poet J. D. McClatchy writes in his poem "My Mammogram":

> . . . the trouble—naturally enough
> Lurking in a useless, overlooked
> Mass of fat and old newspaper stuff
> About matters I regularly mistook
>
> As a horror story for the opposite sex,
> Nothing to do with what at my downtown gym
> Are furtively ogled as The Guy's Pecs.

At the end of his poem, rescued from the bad diagnosis, he wonders, ". . . will I in a decade be back here again, / The diagnosis this time not freakish but fatal?" In an essay McClatchy writes, "I did indeed have a mammogram, and the event's combination of terror and incongruity at once prompted the poem. The procedure itself, less rarely undergone by men than is commonly assumed, raises all sorts of what are now clumsily called 'gender issues.' The staff and doctors, the waiting and examination rooms, the Inspirational Material taped to the walls—everything anticipates a woman's visit. And at the same time, as a man I had no idea of the unholy fear intelligent women endure at regularly scheduled intervals." I thought, *We're all in the same boat, all up the creek, all sinking fast but hoping to rise.* Now I work toward a different trope, know different statistics: every three minutes in the United States another woman is diagnosed with breast cancer. One third of women diagnosed with breast cancer will die of the disease, which means that two thirds won't. Whatever the outcome, we have some time to live. Some of us write and some don't. Some of us go to work, garden, stand on welfare lines, whittle wood, slop paint, dance, sit on stoops in the hot sun worrying about insurance and the cost of dinner. We're teaching, making markets, drafting legislation, and some of us are hanging onto notebooks and slippery pens. We're all living on the margins the best we can.

I read all the published books on breast cancer. The most compelling and frightening ones were personal accounts of suffering, but they didn't help. Dr. Susan Love suggests a reason in her interview: "The books out there are by people who have been through it and so it's their story and they throw in a little medical stuff, which is actually plus-minus accuracy because it's filtered through whatever they got from the one doctor they went to." Before the essays in this book, only Susan Sontag's *Illness as Metaphor* and Oliver Sacks's *A Leg to Stand On*—neither about breast cancer— helped me. Sacks is a medical doctor. He writes about a hiking trip, undertaken alone, and a broken leg. When he crawled from the wilderness for treatment by colleagues unfamiliar with his symptoms, no one believed what he said. As a physician he could see that his leg was in place, but it didn't *feel* like his own, the hitherto unknown symptoms of phantom leg syndrome. Aha! I thought, reading. Breast cancer patients have phantom person syndrome. So then I thought maybe writers with breast cancer can explain why. Maybe they can explain why Audre Lorde, for example, a brilliant writer who died of breast cancer after writing about it in two books, is never identified as a person who died of a disease that was one of her major subjects. Phantom person syndrome.

After surgery, when I went back to work, writers called me on business. To be civil, they asked about my life. When I told them, their responses were surprising. Many had breast cancer. Or they were recovering from treatment. Or they had metastasis and were back in treatment. Taxol, this time. Or acupuncture. But few had told their readers. So I asked each writer to provide a piece for this book. None refused, a major problem when the final cut was required. None of us needed advice. We needed new models of experience. We needed new metaphors. No sinking ships. No heroic victims. In reading their essays and poems, I looked to see how each of us turned our common experience into particular art. Shelters, not oceans. Or, in the reconstructed words of Stevie Smith, "Waving, not drowning."

Conventional wisdom says that suffering ennobles. The most toxic embodiment of this message is Nietzsche's "Whatever doesn't kill us makes us stronger." Cancer patients aren't by definition strong. Nor are we heroes. Cancer patients aren't responsible for our illness or our recoveries, metastases, remissions, or deaths. Conventional wisdom suggests that breast cancer patients have access to death control just as women are supposed to have access to birth control, and if we slip, well, we weren't careful. A friend, after reading her biopsy report, said, "I knew you were a cancer type but I never thought I was." Until now. What now is our human responsibility? Like all the writers gathered together in these pages, we have a human responsibility to live our lives out loud, in our work, as we can.

This book represents a community of workers talking to each other, helping each other, making language serve new imperatives, which is what writers do. We're a community engaged in the same task, making a place of repair where we live. And although we have been bewildered, as all patients are, we love language and our history and assume it will help. In conversation a writer prodded me, "If you're a human being, if you pretend your cancer doesn't exist, you die. If you're a writer and you pretend the experience doesn't exist, do you die? Not physically, but does your art die?" *Living On the Margins* is the answer. As Sandra Spanier wrote of Kay Boyle, we are all "keenly aware of the sentence of mortality that every individual serves." Kay Boyle herself wrote, "You you afraid listen here."

—Hilda Raz
March 1999

Living On
the Margins

Pamela Post

❦

Cancer Says

1993 — Picasso Blue

I HAVE A THREE-INCH SCAR ON MY RIGHT BREAST. It rides a line one and a half inches above the nipple where the intraductal carcinoma was found. Starting in the center of my chest, a radiation burn spirals and grows like the mandala pattern of a galaxy. There are three dotlike permanent tattoos that each day technicians connect with markers to outline the radiation field. They call my favorite marker "Picasso Blue."

I look at myself in the mirror each night as I rub a salve into my burned skin. The multicolored angles and half-circle radiation markings remind me of painted warriors. That is what we are after all—finding the strength to face what might take our life, the courage to march back into battle, patience to wait.

I have not always seen my breast with such detachment. When I removed the bandage three days after the biopsy surgery, I wept at the sight of the black knotted stitches and slash across that tender, pale skin. I felt violated in a way I would not have felt about another part of my body, that I never felt about the emergency appendectomy scar on my abdomen.

Then with the report of cancer there was "wide-excision" surgery, doing just what it claimed. My doctor said the breast would be lifted; it would be smaller but only my husband would know, and if he were worth anything he would not care. But I cared. It had to do with the part of me that first responded to the touch of my teenage boyfriend. It was where my two babies fed and nuzzled and drifted into sleep for the first year of their lives.

I didn't cry again. I thought I would after the wide-excision surgery when I removed the mound of gauze layers taped to me in wide bands, built up like a breast shield. I pulled at each line of tape with deliberation, like peeling an onion. I didn't want the layers to end, but when the only thing left was to lift the last one, I took a deep breath. It was like the moment before diving into the waters of Maine each summer, similar to the breath before I saw my father in his hospital bed, newly diagnosed with lung cancer— the sort of breath you take before something shocks you into not breathing.

My right breast was the size of a fourteen-year-old's. Stormcloud hues of translucent yellow and blue colored the skin as if a watercolorist had been there. My breasts didn't match.

My daughter had come home from college to be with me. She wanted to see for herself. I'm sure she was thinking, as all of our daughters must, *This could happen to me.* I turned to face her. She reached her hand toward me as if bestowing a blessing and pronounced it "fine," just the way she used to comment on my fashion combinations.

As I rub the salve into my skin, I am not embarrassed, nor do I feel diminished by my altered breast. It is a visible daily reminder of my fight and the fight of other women. There are so many of us now, painted in Picasso Blue.

1994 — My Grandmother's Garden

"Is he all tied up?" The man is just coming to; it's late and we're the only ones left in the hospital's day surgery recovery room.

"Is he all tied up?" He calls out again through a haze of anesthesia. The nurses at their rectangular Plexiglas station are finishing up paperwork, ready to go home. Either they can't hear him or they're too tired to pay attention. We're keeping them overtime.

My surgery was delayed two hours. Now I'm sitting in a chair that reminds me of a Barcalounger advertised on TV. I eat saltines and sip ginger ale from a paper cup. If I don't throw it up, they'll send me home. That's the way it goes. This is my fourth surgery since 1993. There was last year's biopsy surgery, followed by wide excision to remove the intraductal carcinoma in situ in my right breast, then this year's biopsy surgery just a month ago. Today they cut out the same cancer in my left breast.

"Is he all tied up?" He is beginning to sound panicky.

"Nurse," I call.

One of them leans around the station. She brushes hair off her forehead. Even in my drugged state, my pores still full of anesthesia, I read her gesture as one of fatigue. She walks toward me with a pan in case I am going to throw up.

"It's not me. It's that man." I point to the hospital bed and I.V. apparatus about twelve feet away from me. "He keeps asking if someone is all tied up."

She goes over to him and looks at his chart. "Leland, is who all tied up?" His eyes are closed. He doesn't seem to hear her. She checks the straps suspending his left leg, which is wrapped in a white plaster cast.

"I don't know, " she says to me. "He had routine leg surgery from a car accident. Nothing was tied, though."

As soon as she is safely in her station he asks, again, "Is he all tied up?"

Suddenly, I know what he is talking about. Every waiting room in the day surgery unit has a television. Earlier in the day, in the registration area where you sign forms that you understand you might die in any number of horrible and unpredictable ways that seem to have nothing at all to do with your surgery, they had *Geraldo* going on the TV screen that hovered, suspended from the ceiling.

Later, after they took all of your clothes and belongings and you were in surgical pants and top with slippers to match, they put you in another room just in time for *Sally Jessy Raphael*. I turned off that television by standing on a chair and pulling out the plug so when a man with at least twenty-five small tumors all over his hands and arms came in, we talked to each other. He was Catholic and prayed to a saint for me. I read to him from one of the notecards I carried, a part from the Ninety-first Psalm about angels having charge over you. Then, when we both got to the pre-surgery room and were put on rolling cots and hooked up to I.V.'s, it was time for a soap opera.

That's when I remember Leland coming in. It was right in the middle of *All My Children.* I was concentrating on my breath, moving it in and out of my belly. It was hard, though, with the television. Every once in a while I'd open my eyes. I remembered a robbery and then I closed my eyes again and used a mantra, "Hummmm, sahhhhhh," the sound of the breath. When they came to take me into surgery, they were tying people up on *All My Children.* Leland must have been watching the same show.

As they wheeled me to the operating room, I began to practice visualization. In a tape I once heard, they said to visualize a garden. So I thought of my grandmother's. I sat on a huge rock down one of its paths. I imagined warm August days as they transferred me from the cot to the cold, metal operating table. The lights above me were harsh. The surgeon's masked face appeared over my head. He said something, but I preferred to close my eyes and watch my grandmother clipping roses from a trellis at the back of the house. Perfect pink roses lying in a cutting basket. This was my last conscious thought.

Leland must have gone into surgery with images of the robbery.

When the nurse comes to take my blood pressure, she says that it is surprisingly good. "It's because of my grandmother's roses," I tell her.

She looks at me quizzically and sticks a thermometer in my mouth. I close my eyes and imagine the lilies-of-the-valley blanketing a huge area just beyond my rope swing. I felt safe going as high as I could, sure that if I fell it would be into the softness of lilies.

"Your little fever is gone," she says, seeming surprised.

"Is he all tied up?"

"Leland," she says moving toward him. "Is who all tied up?" She checks his pulse and blood pressure. She looks exasperated, standing with her hands on her hips.

"It's the TV," I say.

"What?"

"It was the soap opera on in the room before surgery. There was a bank robbery."

"*All My Children?*" she asks. "I see that at home on the days I work the night shift. What happened?"

"I'm not sure. I was trying to meditate."

"Oh." She seems disappointed.

"What do you think of TV in the waiting rooms?" I ask.

"I love television. Since my kids went to college I leave it on all the time," she says.

"Don't you think there is something wrong about a random TV image being the last one you have before surgery?

She shrugs. "It keeps you from thinking about things." She looks at the clock. "How do you feel?"

"I'm fine," I say. I'm still mostly protected from pain by the drugs. I'm not thinking about things either.

"You can go home now. I'll call your husband." She leads me into a room and hands me the bag with my clothes. It hurts to raise my left arm, and I have to get out of the hospital robe and into my shirt. It's winter and I also have to find a way to pull on my boots. I manage it, although I realize that I have my stirrup pants on backwards.

After I'm dressed I wait in a wheelchair by the door in the day surgery unit. It will be a long wait. My husband has not responded well to my cancer. After the first biopsy, I read him the statistics of breast cancer pulling women from life, sometimes just for a while, sometimes forever. He sat unmoved as I wept over the numbers. Today, he acts as if I'm here for a broken arm. He'll take his time in coming for me. Another thing I can't spend much time thinking about.

I don't see any harm in it, so I wheel myself over to Leland's bed. His I.V. looks almost finished. He's a nice-looking man, mid-forties with some gray at his temples. "Is he all tied up?" he asks again.

I say, "Yes. All tied up and taken care of. The police are in charge and even the robbers are better off. They needed to be caught for the good of their karma." I almost laugh. It must be the anesthesia. I've never even thought about karma before.

"Listen, Leland," I say. "There is a place. My grandmother's garden. It's scented with honeysuckle. Evening primrose gleams like yellow gold." I tell him about the pathways of crushed white shells that lead you to its center: an old stone birdbath. I say that in that garden everything grows perfectly, and that if you sit there for any length of time you heal perfectly, too.

I have made that part up but suddenly believe it. I close my eyes and can almost feel the wound on my breast healing shut. I don't know how long I sit like that with my eyes closed.

"Lilacs," Leland says.

"Yes. Lilacs in the spring. White and lavender and deep purple ones."

The nurse comes for me. My husband is waiting downstairs. He will be indifferent to my ordeal. I expect it. I'll have to go back to that garden. I'll find my grandmother who loved me and would have hoped to spare me all of life's pain.

"Leland," I say as the nurse wheels me away. "If you can smell the lilacs you'll wake up soon."

1996 — Billie

The nurse calls the woman Billie. We are separated by curtains, one that could wrap around my hospital bed following its train-track ceiling route, and one that could wrap around hers. Long and drapelike they hang heavy, dull-checkered, and thick between us. At night, as I am awakened for medicine or vital sign tabulations or by pain that roars through my chest and back, I see late movies flickering in the darkness above my curtain. Billie moans. I can hear it over or maybe under the actors' voices. Her broken sounds are aching and some part of me is too sick to care, but another part wonders what hurts her so much.

In the morning light, I think about Billie's crying and guess that her pain is, as it is for me and every other human being, cumulative. There is the wound or operation or illness that hits our bodies. And there is heartache in its various forms woven in and out of our souls. Which does she cry for? Which pain is it? Or is it both?

I don't cry, but I have pain, too. The most obvious, a lost and reconstructed breast, with a jagged scar running down my back that looks like a random, thoughtless slicing. Gauze and tape cover wounds and drain sites. Some sources of pain I can feel and others I cannot yet, still numbed by severed nerves and medications strong enough to take me up and out of this hospital room.

Then there is my divorce. So far, my children and I have kept moving on, but here I am immobile and I fear the hurt and abandonment that circle above my bed, waiting to settle their talons and weight on me.

In the morning, a nurse calls her and Billie answers. She sounds like one of my students, a seventh-grade boy who reminded me from the start of a bird: black, lustrous, delicate, skittish. I worked with him carefully, as if one wrong move or word and he'd take flight. Twice a week I'd put my finger out for him to land on and hold my breath to see if he'd stay. Week after week. Before this operation we were into our second year, and he'd found his perch. Billie's voice is soft, uncertain, tentative, as if it might not hold in the air. But at night it fills the room.

I am silent. My crying sticks in me, just as if they'd put their dressings and gauze and tape to hold my tears in place. The tubes coming out of me do not drain despair and the tubes going in bring healing only for my body—nothing deeper. When I talk on the phone or to a nurse or visitor, I describe the beauty of the flowers sent to me: the pink begonia in its sandalwood basket, the dozen white roses arranged with eucalyptus and heather, the vase from the Brattle Square Florist holding a summer's garden of lilies, iris, and sunflowers. I don't talk about how the pain medication makes me so sick that they have to alternate morphine with Compazine, or how much it hurts just to move in bed, my back cut and filled with tubes. My new breast pulls and aches where my own had been. I don't think about the surgeries I've had in the past although my doctor told me that I held my body rigidly, as if I knew when each cut was coming. My body remembered.

On the second day Billie speaks to me. She says in her whispery voice that barely makes it through the curtain that she is sorry she had the television on all night; the nurse has told her that it kept me awake. The pain is so great, she says, that the only thing that helps is to watch the movies. She sounds matter-of-fact, as if she too has trouble talking about what hurts when the sun is up. I say that if it's the only thing that helps her, keep the television on. I say that my daughter can bring me earplugs.

She seems grateful. I can hear it in her voice gathering itself up like a bird taking flight. She confesses that the pain squeezes at her until she is almost passing out. I hear how they started with cutting off her toes, a few at a time and then cut off her leg first right above the ankle. She describes how they keep coming back to do more and then this last time they took it right below the knee, and now they say that they don't know if they have to be going back again. Her words dip down. "I haven't been home in six months," she says. I imagine her crumpled down in bed, her body fading with her voice.

I say that I am sorry. That I have lost things, too. I don't know what home is anymore. My husband is gone. My children are grown and away at school. My body aches, too. Pain settles, perches, nests, reproduces, and I try not to let it go too deeply in.

I want to get up to see Billie now that we've talked, but I'm hooked to too many tubes and I don't even know if my arms will lift me into a sitting position or if my legs still work. Morphine drips into me, making me think I can walk, but I can't figure out how to rid myself of the catheter and lingering epidural lines.

That night she has the sound all the way off and I am grateful, but when they wake me to take my blood pressure I still hear her crying. I ask the night nurse when I'll be loose from so much tubing and she says by tomorrow night I'll be able to get up to use the bathroom and the antibiotic and pain medication drips can roll along with me on their metal stand.

And it is true. By the time Billie starts her crying the next night I have already been up twice and I know exactly how far my legs will carry me. I can get to her.

She starts her wail way down low, and I push the button to raise my bed. Its whirring sound is drowned out by her crying. In this upright position, I can see out the window. Mission Hill bathes in the light of a full moon so bright that the colors of the houses are visible. Sitting, I can smell the sweetness of the roses on my windowsill, and I breathe them in as if they'll give me strength. I begin to hoist myself up on my right elbow. I, who have loved the strength in my arms from working out, find it hard now to make this simple move, but before I know it I am sitting up and pulling my legs over to dangle from the bed. The I.V.'s in my arm will move with me—in fact, their stand adds support as I edge myself down to the floor and shuffle around the drapes to her bed.

Billie is sitting up. Everything is dark except for her sheets and the layers and layers of moon-white gauze wrapped around the stump of her leg. Her skin is a glossy brown, her hair tied back in a dark bandanna. She has on her own nightgown, a soft navy cotton one. She's probably sixty; she looks like someone's grandma.

She rocks herself back and forth, holding onto her bandaged leg as if it were a baby she's cradling. Her moans and tears mix together so that my heart almost breaks now that I can see her. I get myself up on the bed beside her with the help of my pole. She doesn't seem surprised. I come to her bandaged too and without speaking she keeps rocking.

I rub her back in unison with her rocking so that we're both moving together and she tells me that the pain doesn't seem to stop. All these operations. I feel her pain and it opens me up as much as the surgeon's knife and this time what comes out are my feelings. I can't stand it either, all these surgeries. My chest begins to heave; we keep moving together as if we're all one motion, her rocking leg, my rubbing arm, our sobbing throats. She says that she's losing her home because she can't work and I suddenly feel my house empty. It's just another divorced couple's house on the market, but I cry for all the fires in the fireplace and family dinners at the table that will be too big for anyplace I will ever live again.

She cries for the pain and I rock along with her. I tell her that I've never known such burning and pulling at my flesh. She'll never be the same, she says, and I know what she means and then we don't talk. My sobbing grows and overtakes hers. Billie rocks years of tears out of me just as surely as if she were cradling me in her arms instead of her leg. We do this for the next two nights, as illicit as lovers forbidden to meet. I give her touch that soothes her and she takes me to a place in the darkness, alongside her grief where I too can cry.

But in the morning, at the residents' early rounds, I am brave and strong and take it all with courage. People like me to behave that way. I like it, too. I thought that's the way it had to be until I found Billie and the nights and finally a way to let go of sorrow and rage and hurt that kept me raw and empty inside.

During the day the clusters of residents and doctors and nurses tend to our bodies, but at night Billie and I tend to our souls.

1997—Cancer Says

I lie in bed once again at the time of the winter solstice. It is the darkest day of the year. I stare at the candles on my grandmother's wicker table that became my altar when I first had cancer. I used to burn a fat blue candle with a drifting smell of lavender, a white taper in a silver candlestick, and a votive in a gilded, star-cut container with light flickering out, as if to a night sky. I have not lit them since my surgery. Over the altar hangs a Matisse sketch of a nude with full breasts, thick heavy nipples. Further up on the wall is a New Mexico cross, two sticks fastened at their center with garlic cloves and dried red peppers.

In the darkness I hear "Silent Night" from the stereo downstairs. My son and a friend from college are stringing lights on the tree. We always used multicolored bulbs, but the boys went out a few hours ago and bought five strands of tiny, starlike white lights. When he was small I taught my son that stars were for wishing. He now says in his stage of questioning God that while others pray, he looks for a star. I know he is afraid. Tomorrow or the next day we'll have the pathology report. His friend downstairs lost his mother to breast cancer; as he watches me, I wonder how much he thinks of his mother. How much does my son think of his friend's mother, buried six years?

This is my second mastectomy, my seventh and eighth surgery. Seventh, the mastectomy itself, eighth the reconstruction, one following the other with a half-hour break to change "teams" as if my body were a playing field.

This is the first time I have really understood I have cancer. With the original surgery five years ago, denial's seed pushed up and produced a sheltering tree so vast that when I looked to the sky I could see only bits of lacy blue. I felt little threat to my life. Instead I focused mostly on the plight of women with breast cancer. I saw us as sisters: bruised, cut, stitched, and marred. Then when the suspicious mammogram, the confirmed malignancy, the surgery and subsequent radiation occurred again a year later, I sat under the shade of the tree and looked around, talking about the other patients but saying little about myself. With the third surgery two years later, they took my breast altogether. That surgery knocked me down. It was winter and through the bare sinewy branches I saw a stormcloud sky. Gunmetal. Fast moving. A sky full of tears. Today, I'm laid out flat recovering from another surgery—another breast. The tree above me is still bare; the winter sky is dull, unmoving, a ceaseless gray with no puffs of clouds or streaks of sunlight. I am totally exposed to whatever it might do: snow, sleet, blow a northeaster hard for days.

A week ago, after I woke up from the surgery, I wondered if it was my breast they had taken. Had they removed my heart? Stitched my mouth shut? I had nothing to say. I knew the routine of recovery: the drain sites with their plastic tubes and suction cup containers, the lengthy knifing across my back marking the taking of the latissimus dorsi to make a breast. I knew how long before I'd be able to walk, that morphine made me sick but that I could tolerate doses of synthetic heroin. I remembered the casings they put on my legs to prevent clots, the plastic filling up with air every few minutes and then deflating like a slow breath taken in, held, and let out. I knew to order puddings and tea with extra milk. I knew what to do, but I no longer knew what to say.

The news comes that I have slipped through cancer's narrowing noose once again. I do not have invasive cancer, and for days I am lifted out of my mourning. I come downstairs and sit by the tree; the lights burn through my melancholy. Each ornament is full of meaning—the ones my children made long ago from pine cones, yearly cross-stitched Christmas sentiments from an aunt, the hand-blown glass balls friends have given me each year. I ask my son to turn "The Messiah" to full volume to fill the house. When I was growing up, my father used to sing it every year with a chorus. I close my eyes and hear his bass part, the one he rehearsed in the bathroom each morning while he shaved. The smell of molasses and sugar drifts through the house. My daughter is home now, and she bakes gingerbread men the way I used to and frosts them with white pants, green shoes, yellow hair. They have cinnamon drops for eyes, so that they look like clowns. We laugh. We all rejoice.

A few days after Christmas, though, I don't get out of bed. I don't raise the shades. I lie there until the visiting nurse comes to change my dressing. Once she's gone, I'm back under the covers. I'm so still inside I wonder if I'm alive. My spirit, I realize, is as scarred as my body. Have I gone through all of this finally to give up?

At the end of the week, the silence that has wrapped itself around me is pushed away by loud voices. They're my own. Screams I'd stuffed back not with a fist but with a smile; not with a gag but with my own refusal to pay attention. Pain drones right through the center of the wails. It shapes itself from the hours waiting for pathology reports. The first time, when I hadn't heard for eight days, I dressed to go to work. I called the doctor's office when I had my coat on. The nurse said the results had just come through and the doctor needed to talk to me. "Don't go to work," she said, and I sat by the phone for the next hour. When I think of waiting and bad news now, I see myself in that navy wool coat sitting alone by the phone waiting to be told I had cancer. Pain shapes itself from the repeated slicing of my palest flesh; from the mammograms in those rooms where other women glided in and out, exchanging the "johnny" for their own clothes as I sat, pulling the cotton gown close around my body, and they called me in again, first for another view and then a magnification and the cheerful technician who eventually couldn't even look at me and became grimly silent herself except to say, "Move in closer.... Lift your right arm.... Hold your breath."

I think now it's as if I've been holding my breath for five years. I gasp in mouthfuls.

My scream carries through the house. My keening climbs the attic stairs, settles into the depths of the basement, sweeps through the rooms. This pain penetrates the walls so that when I've moved, this house will remember not only my beautiful children as they grew from toddlers to young adults, but it will have recorded what I finally felt.

An explosion has occurred in me, and fury snakes into the air. I want to rip out all the I.V.'s I've had since 1993; I want to snatch the scalpels from the surgeons' hands and plunge them into the earth where they'll cut no more. I would return my muscles to my back and take a club to the radiation machines maneuvering into place to kill my cells. If I could, I'd try to find my lovely pink nipples in the midst of my discarded flesh and then drug all the doctors with an anesthesia as strong as mine—let them be gone from this earth for eight-hour stretches.

But the doctors were as kind as anyone could have hoped. I'm not mad at them. It's not God either, for I do not believe God punishes. It's loss I throw my rage at. It rolls along, gathering new parts of my life. It circles me, waiting for the kill, for I am now so vulnerable. My breasts cut from me. My husband's desertion and divorce, my children grown, my house to be sold. I scream to scatter loss. I swing my arms out in the air, throw back my head and yell to stop, please, please to stop.

As the days pass, I feel calmer, and oddly, I return to where I began five years before—feeling the pain of millions of women with breast cancer. I think of my friend Susan, whose spine crumbled after cancer spread to her bones and the woman who had her first child aborted at three months when they discovered her breast full of tumors. I ask for healing. For me. For them.

Cancer takes your life and changes it, transforms it forever, and sometimes, as it does for me today, gives it back. Cancer then says to take up your broken self once again and, if you are able, fashion something even better than what you had before—"before my visits began," cancer says.

Maxine Kumin

❦

Off

TWO WEEKS POST-OP; FINALLY, I FEEL READY TO reflect on my breast cancer and the subsequent surgery.

Last June, a routine annual gyn exam. That same day, as always, a mammogram. About a week later, my gynecologist called me at home. She and I have a somewhat special relationship, as we are both horse fanatics and annually must exchange snapshots and anecdotes before we proceed to speculum and pelvic exam. In fact, I had seen her at the big three-day driving show in Vermont a few months back and was thrilled that she had, unbeknownst to me, witnessed my gelding's clean traversal of a twenty-obstacle cones course. She told me then that she had had a mastectomy three months before that, was back to her practice in one week, and felt she had adjusted to her new state of affairs. I didn't offer sympathy but congratulations. Surgery in time is a narrow escape. She'd had wonderful luck; we both acknowledged it.

There are five tiny dots on the mammogram. The radiologist recommends redoing it in six months, but I don't think we ought to wait that long, was what she said.

Given her history, I thought. I thought, breast cancer is not my karma. I'm more likely to get killed bouncing out of the cart (I had already racked up once that year, driving my three-year-old, who reared, caught her hip under a shaft, fell, and tossed me out on my helmeted head).

I'm suggesting you have this area biopsied. The surgeon who

operated on me is pretty talented at finding these calcifications. Let's get it out and see what pathology says.

Ultra-conservative, I thought. But I trusted her. I said yes.

One must always see the surgeon face to face first. Another appointment, another trip an hour up the interstate. I was prepared to like him, as I would have been prepared to like whomever she recommended. He was icily correct. No verbal chisel at my disposal was going to penetrate that rectitude.

What are the chances this is just a calcium deposit?

I have been doing this procedure for thirty years, he told me. And I have been wrong exactly twice.

My antennae quivered. It was pretty clear he didn't like to be questioned. Nevertheless, I made the appointment for a biopsy to be done on an out-patient basis.

No word was spoken to prepare me for this procedure. I had not yet seen the Susan Love book; afterwards, I thought how much mental gnashing I might have been spared if I had read her chapter on biopsy ahead of time. A lamb to the slaughter, I lay down for the first injection of lidocaine, followed by the insertion of a thin wire into the presumptive five-dotted spot. Up then for another mammogram. Down again for repositioning of wire. Up again, down again. The surgeon never addressed me as human. He is intent on doing it right, I told myself. Four tries and he was satisfied. Partially dressed, I walked to the elevator, went up one flight to Day Surgery, entered the operating room. A very fat nurse introduced herself. It was clear that her bunions hurt; she walked as little as possible.

A lot of fussing about ensued to position me for the comfort and visibility of the surgeon. My arm was tied up behind my head. A grounding wire for the electrocautery lay across my body. The surgeon was not happy with the arrangement; he needed to sit in order to cut. More pumping table to new height, arm dragging behind in excruciating posture, finally elevated to a bearable level. Lidocaine. Scalpel. Cautery. Distinct smell of burning flesh, for which I was not prepared; a barbecue, lacking the sauce. Scalpel. Cautery. Lidocaine.

I went inward as far as I could, concentrating on relaxing various outlying muscles, not easy in view of my chronic rotator cuff tendinitis from lugging winter water buckets. In the ensuing hour and a half the surgeon spoke only once. "Tedious, tedious," he sighed.

It's tedious for me, too, I thought. And I'm not getting paid for it.

At last he held up a glistening plug of tissue the length of my little finger and twice as thick. This was sent down to be x-rayed to be certain he had gotten the entire cluster of calcifications.

Silence during the wait for verification. He and the fat nurse chatted minimally. Of course he called her Beth and of course she called him Dr. X. I was mercifully, or unmercifully, ignored. Word arrived that the biopsy was complete.

As he began to sew me up, in an effort to break the silence I asked, "How many stitches are you taking?"

"I don't know! Twenty-seven! You can tell all your friends you had twenty-seven stitches!"

What had I done? Whatever it was, it wasn't politically correct, it seemed.

As he prepared to leave (I was still prone, arm still held captive), I tried to ask him what sort of follow-up procedure would take place.

She'll tell you, he said, jerking his head in the nurse's direction. He didn't exactly leave; he fled.

A week later, he called. You have noninvasive intraductal carcinoma.

What does that mean?

It means you have three choices. You can do nothing. You can take tamoxifen. Or you can have a mastectomy. You'll have to come in and let me explain this to you.

Another trip north. I called his office and made an appointment. In the meantime, I said I wanted a copy of the pathology report.

I have to get Dr. X's permission for that, the secretary informed me.

I don't think so. I think legally I am entitled to that information. Please see that it is sent to me.

I still have to get Doctor's permission.

I hung up.

Two days later, a one-sentence letter from Dr. X reiterating that he would have to talk to me face to face to interpret the report. Two days after that, just as I was reaching a fast boil, the path report arrived.

By then I had acquired *Dr. Susan Love's Breast Book.* It told me everything he had not. Also, by then I had done some networking. Several of my friends had already been through this maze and I followed their various threads. One thing I knew: I would have to go elsewhere for my follow-up, whatever form it took.

I am ashamed to say that I lied to Dr. X. At the highly touted appointment, which lasted less than five minutes, he began (tediously, tediously) to draw a diagram of a duct. I pulled out the Susan Love book, opened it to her diagrams of the various stages, and said, "I've read about this. Do you know this wonderful book?"

He grew more terse. My gynecologist told me afterward that he "has a thing about Susan Love." Like Oedipus who begs Jocasta not to enquire further, I did not enquire further.

But I lied. I said when I had made my decision I would get back to him. This time, I was the one in flight.

I can't talk to him, I told my gyn. I want to go to the Faulkner.

Susan Love founded the Faulkner Breast Center. She then went on to establish a similar facility in Los Angeles. The Center was then staffed almost entirely by women, women the ages of my daughters. Crisp, professional, caring, and above all, female. I never looked back.

The Faulkner Hospital in Boston lies two and a half hours away in the other direction, through horrible traffic. One thing about living in the country: it spoils you for city driving. Just going "downtown," two miles in summer, when tourists add about 1,500 souls to our established population of 2,000, feels like a penance. All the angled parking spaces in front of the little grocery store are taken! But I grueled through the snarl for a first appointment with Kathleen Strah, a surgeon who looks to be about thirty. She still has braces on her teeth. Well, maybe she's thirty-five. She is the mother of a toddler, commutes into the city from Harvard, Massachusetts, and is wonderfully direct in manner.

We agreed that there was no immediate urgency about my breast and that I could meet my several reading and residency commitments that fall. We scheduled the surgery for the week before Thanksgiving. In the meantime, I managed to tear a disc in my neck undertaking that most banal of autumn tasks, raking leaves. It was hideously slow to heal and I was still wearing a neck collar and enduring considerable chronic pain by the time of my surgery.

Everyone was cheerful and considerate. I was permitted to wear the collar right into pre-op and awakened with it in place after the two-and-a-half-hour cutting. Moreover, I was encouraged to bring my own very soft pillow with me in place of the hospital pillows, which turned out to be an excellent idea.

Looking back, I think the toughest part of the procedure was the thirty minutes my husband, Victor, and I sat out in the hospital parking lot that gray November morning, killing time until the appointed hour. We had departed New Hampshire at dawn; I of course was breakfastless (nothing after midnight), which never improves my disposition. The night before, trying not to be histrionic, I dictated a list of where I wanted my various horses to go in case I expired under the knife (not very likely, I acknowledged). He was terrific about it, but then he is a very sane and balanced person and he's had long years of practice in smoothing me down when I grow irrational.

At the Faulkner, surgery begins with an early-morning admittance, much kinder, I think, than the olden days when you entered that domain the night before and slept only fitfully in a strange bed while awaiting the unknown. Victor took my wedding ring, earrings, and watch as well as my winter coat. I was shepherded down a long corridor to a dressing room, given a plastic bag in which to deposit everything I was wearing, and then conveyed in johnny and robe and throw-away slippers to a gurney. Several of us were stacked side by side like birch logs awaiting the sawyer, but even this difficult passage from sentience to unconsciousness was lightened by two bantering aides and a television set. One of the aides tapped into my vein and slipped me a lovely Demerol Mickey. I was not awake for the rest of the journey into the O.R.

By mid-afternoon I was conscious, in a small but private room on the seventh floor with one big window overlooking a still-green slope of hillside that leads to the Arnold Arboretum. It was a user-friendly view, one I came to appreciate at dawn, midday, sunset, and, with the twinkling of various street lights, in the dark hours as well.

I was encouraged to get up, use the private bathroom on my own at twilight that same day and was gratified to have my plumbing gradually return to normal. The amputation was very lightly bandaged with gauze pads held in place by strips of not-very-sticky tape. These pieces began falling off almost immediately and by the next morning I had to face in the mirror what looked like a chainsaw-rendered incision. A nurse stood by me for that first peek; she was so matter-of-fact that I would have been ashamed to flail about and react badly. (For a few weeks what I mostly felt was recoil, sympathy for my wounded self, and a slight admixture of horror over what had been done.) Dr. Strah assured me that first evening and on the next day that the incision looked terrific—*gorgeous* was the word she used, then amended, gorgeous from a surgeon's point of view. The weekend was upon us; a Dr. Macintosh would be covering for her on Saturday and Sunday. Chances were good I'd go home on Monday, as soon as the drains came out. The drains, two doughnut-shaped rubber gizmos, hung from my nightgown. Plastic tubing from them ran into the incision to carry away the blood and serum of the cut. Because my chest wall was undisturbed—no breaking and sawing of bones—there wasn't any serious discomfort, though I turned a brilliant black and blue all over the area of my now-absent breast. Orders had been left for Percocet every three or four hours, though, and because of my neck I was happy to take advantage of what was offered. Floating up out of my skin on Percocet, I understood the release, the euphoria the addict experiences, demands, will kill for.

Because Victor had made every round trip to the hospital with me, I insisted, now that the surgery was behind us, that he give himself a break over the weekend. Besides, we have no barn help on Saturdays and Sundays, which limits our mobility. He called me Saturday night and asked, "Well, how did you like Dr. Macintosh? What'd he have to say?"

"I have news for you, honey," I told him. "*She's* black."

And stunning. And well-dressed. We have a lawyer daughter who has that same impeccably groomed, don't-try-me demeanor, the perfect, chicly tailored suit softened with something like a Dior scarf at the neck or an exquisitely configured lapel pin.

I have to say how much I enjoyed looking at these young professionals, how much pleasure I took from their obvious success at invading the final male bastion of medical privilege. We talked a bit about my generation's struggle to break into the male-dominated academic world. Dr. Macintosh told me she was one of six children, each out now in the world doing his or her own thing, one teaching, another a lawyer, and so on. A real morale booster. I thought how it would have been with icy Dr. X in the north country and was grateful once again that I had followed my instinct.

"Oh, that Dr. Macintosh!" said Dr. Strah on Monday when I commented on the fashion figure she cut, "She makes it so tough for the rest of us to keep up with her."

I thought she was keeping up quite well in her Liz Claiborne houndstooth check pantsuit, or what I could see of it beneath the white doctor's coat as she bent to remove one drain. The other was still filling with fluid; we agreed I would stay one more day. I found I was in no hurry to leave the hospital, the push-button conveniences, the congenial nurses whose life stories I had already appropriated. The food was unseasoned, steam-table bland, but Victor had laid in a supply of fresh fruit, pretzels, and other goodies. I walked around a lot that final twenty-four hours but I also lay in bed a lot leafing through magazines, admiring the view from my window, a view I had come to feel quite proprietary about with its best beech tree and the remnants of a stone wall, well repaired. I realized how grateful I was to have the surgery behind me, to have a gorgeous chain-saw slash across the area where I had once had a left breast, to give in to this mild melancholy and lassitude, to be surrounded by floral arrangements with tender notes attached.

This, the winter of 1993-94, was as far as I got in recording my impressions. I do remember that the prosthetic fitter came to the hospital with her measuring tape and provided me with some soft synthetic material to stuff into my bra when I dressed to leave. I was grateful to don that stretched-out old bra; my spirits were further buoyed when I saw in the mirror that nothing about my appearance had changed. I think that at first the impulse is to disguise at all costs the fact that you have lost a breast. It took me several months to get over that instinctual response. It took even longer—possibly a full year—for me to come to terms with this absence. The skin under the scar has no feeling of its own; the nerves have been removed along with the mammary tissue. At first the brain struggles to reconnect. I kept feeling my missing nipple. It tingled as in arousal. It itched. It screamed, I am still here! as in the well-documented phantom limb syndrome. I had to force myself to run my hand, ever so lightly, over my newly flat plane. Alicia Ostriker had said, Make friends with your scar. Touch it a lot. This was hard to do. I still shunned my sliced-clean chest as an ugliness, an unpleasant sensation.

When I went back to the Faulkner for my six-weeks checkup, Shirley the Fitter met me again. It's funny, the things that stay in my memory. Wearing shorts and tights, she was charmingly unprofessional in appearance, all business when I stripped to be measured. My insurance paid to have one bathing suit and two bras modified for a prosthesis. When the box came it contained various gizmos that would permit the wearer, six months post-op, to plaster the prosthesis directly to her concavity. There were ointments to attach, emollients to detach, an eyebrow pencil for marking exactly where the attachment should go, a dozen skin pads to stick in place, and a booklet of instructions. Dutifully I kept this treasure trove in my bureau for a whole year. Eventually I chucked it out, saving only the eyebrow pencil for which there might be some future use.

That summer, into my old at-home black bathing suit I sewed a black shoulder pad. I, who had always disrobed with aplomb among friends at the pond, found I was reluctant to swim in the buff with company now that I had only one breast. I also found it a nuisance to wear a bra and circumvented the issue about 90 percent of the time by adopting loose-fitting tops. Another ploy was to acquire two or three vests, one a lacy white, another a sporty print. Present fashion makes it easy to disappear the disappearance, as it were.

I never went back to the Faulkner after my initial checkup; it was easier simply to return to the care of my gyn, who told me she couldn't be bothered with bras either. In addition to schooling her two thoroughbreds she has now taken up scuba diving. She's only a year or two away from retirement, and then she plans to get into carriage driving. I really feel that she saved my life.

Two years have now passed. Blue Cross/Blue Shield permitted me to acquire a second prosthesis, so now I can keep one permanently in my best bathing suit. Since I seldom feel called upon to wear a bra, my two white nylon 36A's should last me a dozen years. I have finally made friends with my scar and can almost admire my naked pre-adolescent self on that side.

We are an ever enlarging women's club, we one- or no-breasters. I recently sat on a writers' panel with three other mastectomized women, all of us willing to discuss our experiences, our lymph nodes, radiations and/or chemos. How fortunate I was to have made the decision opting for a total mastectomy with no further treatment over a lumpectomy and six weeks of radiation! When the pathologist examined the tissue from the operation, she found a second area of intraductal cancer under the areola, where it would have lain undetected, Dr. Strah thought, for another two years. Then there's my good friend Lois, who had the same diagnosis as I. She chose the lumpectomy route. In the course of radiation an undocumented error was made by the technicians. Her lung on that side was burned, reducing her respiratory capacity by one third. Forever, that is. The radiation also gave rise to lymphedema of the upper arm, a fat arm she will have to live with presumably forever. But worst of all, the fatigue from radiation dragged her into the lower depths. A psychiatric social worker, she was barely able to hang on to her practice, spending every available break between patients lying down, trying to recover the energy needed to carry on.

My older brothers as late adolescents used to tell an off-color joke about a tailor who was measuring a client for a suit jacket. I don't remember the joke, only the gesture: Oh, you don't want a breast pocket? I'll rub it out.

Rubbed out figuratively and literally, I am happy to be here.

Judith Hall

❦

A Design Upon Us

And yet you will *weep and know why.*
—*Gerard Manley Hopkins*

IN 1811, WHEN FANNY BURNEY DESCRIBED HER breast cancer in a letter to her sister Esther, she composed the earliest record of a rudimentary mastectomy, and her letter eventually passed into the documentary history of western medicine. She noted symptoms, the unsymptomatic pain in her breast; and she noted her French husband M. d'Arblay's concern. "The most sympathising of Partners, however, was more disturbed: not a start, not a wry face, not a movement that indicated pain was unobserved..."

After months of uncertainty and repugnance, and finally, catapulted by anxiety, she consulted M. Dubois, the Empress Josephine's surgeon. He asked if she had felt much pain when her son was born, if she had screamed or cried; she said yes. "I told him, it had not been possible to do otherwise," which, she wrote, seemed to be the answer he wanted, but "what terrible inferences were here to be drawn!" M. Dubois made a preliminary diagnosis, but since he was preoccupied with the Empress's complaints, he passed Fanny Burney on to his colleague, Dominique-Jean Larrey. Baron de Larrey was First Surgeon to Napoleon and Surgeon-in-Chief to the Grande Armée. He agreed to perform her mastectomy before leaving for the Russian front. Fanny Burney talked to him a little of her husband, her "too sympathising" husband. She wanted to protect him, if possible, and asked the surgeon not to mention her imminent ordeal, at least not until it was over. They debated this, but the surgeon seems to have agreed.

Then he said that she would have a few hours' warning before he came to her Paris house and did the surgery in her salon.

Fanny Burney's first novel, an epistolary novel, *Evelina; or, The History of a Young Lady's Entrance into the World*, created a sensation when it appeared in London in 1778. Burney was twenty-five. Ten years of diary-writing were an ad-hoc apprenticeship but so were her correspondences with her sisters. The language of these letters was robust and ebullient, because these messages were private. Her novel captured this vivacity and was also admired as a first glimpse of the "young lady's" point of view. Burney learned, from her sister Maria's letters, how painful it could be to negotiate a first London season; and how a young lady's life could be altered by the language of a fan.

London hostesses competed with one another to discover the anonymous author of *Evelina*. When Fanny Burney claimed the novel as her own, Dr. Samuel Johnson impulsively kissed her hand. Dr. Johnson was not impulsive as a rule. Fanny Burney recorded the kiss in her diary and the smear of butter that he left on her hand.

Thirty-three years later, living in Paris, she does not compose in her diary her surgery. She does not mention the prognosis, the doctor's office, or the time she waited before surgery; her twenty-five-minute surgery. She passes over it. "When I was sufficiently recovered for travelling, after a dreadful operation..." She describes her journey with her son to England. Napoleon's war threatened him with the draft. She writes from such a distance, in retrospect, that she might as well be remembering an unpleasant dinner party without music, offered by the wrong hostess. Some of her biographers, up until the middle of the twentieth century, followed her example and did not mention her breast cancer at all. Why was it easier for her to write her sister about the surgery than to write to herself—a more intimate audience, surely—in her diary?

*

To Esther, Fanny Burney confided the moment when both M. Dubois and M. Larrey arrived, and in their wide shadow, "seven men in black." One gave her wine. The others, later, together, held her down during surgery. The wine and the men comprised her anesthesia. Old mattresses were thrown into the middle of her salon. Her maid and two nurses began to cry, and M. Dubois ordered the women out.

> No, I cried, let them stay! "Qu'elles restent!" This occasioned a little dispute that re-animated me—The Maid, however, & one of the nurses ran off—I charged the other to approach, & she obeyed. M. Dubois now tried to issue his commands en militaire, but I resisted all that was resistable.

M. Dubois covered her face with his cambric handkerchief, but she saw him through the finely woven cloth. Her surgeon's face was ashen gray. She saw "the glitter of polished Steel—I closed my Eyes."

Then the silence in the small salon frightened her. She writes of the silence, and the signs she imagined the doctors made to one another. She heard M. Larrey ask, "Qui me tiendra ce sein?" ["Who will hold the breast for me?"] When no one replied, Fanny Burney feared "they imagined the whole breast infected." She opened her eyes and saw, through the handkerchief, M. Dubois draw a line and then a circle over one entire breast. "I started up, threw off my veil, & in answer to the demand 'Qui me tiendra ce sein' cried 'C'est moi, Monsieur!' & I held my hand under it, and explained the nature of my sufferings..."

The surgeons ignored her intervention. One of them replaced the handkerchief. Then Fanny Burney described the incision; the angle of it and the flesh cut; the nerves; the pain; the air on the wound and the edges of the wound. Her eyes shut: "they felt as if hermetically shut, & so firmly closed, that the Eyelids seemed indented to the Cheeks..." The surgeon moved rapidly, scraping the breast bone of malignancies, "attom after attom," and she added, "My dearest Esther, not for Weeks, but for Months I could not speak of this terrible business without nearly again going through it!"

Why was it easier for Fanny Burney to write her sister about her mastectomy than to write about it in her diary? If she wanted to divulge her experience, spill it on the page, and divulge her raw, confused feelings, couldn't she have done this in her diary? To write is to embody some vital blend of event and imagining. Perhaps alone, writing in her diary, Burney lost some sense of proportion. She faltered. The event could not be "recollected in tranquility," not the palpable sensation of wounds. Alone, she kept the trauma at a great distance, tiny, almost out of mind, but not quite out of mind, because she was safer, guarded, if she kept the trauma (she kept it; she controlled it) in her mind, but tiny: "When I was sufficiently recovered for travelling, after a dreadful operation..." It is noted—how dreadful—and the writer rushes past.

When she tried to articulate her experience, again Fanny Burney found the memory too vivid, overwhelming. She wrote to Esther, "not for Weeks, but for Months I could not speak of this terrible business without nearly again going through it!" She could not speak of it. A listener, a human presence watching and hearing her, was not the consolation she might have expected. It was not the reply, the content or fact of the reply, that troubled her. Any listener, whole and wholly separate from herself, was not tolerable, even if the person served as mirror or witness to her pain. Fanny Burney could not speak to herself or to someone else or hear a "too sympathetic" reply.

Now the value of writing to her absent sister Esther seems more clear. She will tell someone, but someone who is not in the room. Imagining her sister, she is bolstered enough to proceed and sustained enough to linger in her memory. She writes, conjuring her sister, but only as needed, half-consciously. She controls each element of confession, writing scene after scene of her body in the most awful extremity.

Is it possible to write and not go "through it" again? Perhaps, if the writing is divorced from bodily imagination, if it is some fantasy of abstract reportage; if it is a pure intelligence. But that is not what Burney does. The idea of an absent beloved sister stabilizes and then enables the writer's imaginings. She blends her prognosis, her surgery, the facts of her case, with the detailed complications— interpretations, denials, flights—of her particular brain.

When she finished her difficult composition, Burney could have leaned back in her Empire chair, rereading her letter, and had one of several responses to it. She might have felt surprised reading a simple sequence on the page. However well formed, the grammar and narrative coherence would be a strangely partial translation of her complicated memories. She recognized herself, though, and in her solitary recognition scene, she began to accept, a little, what had happened to her. In this moment, the letter serves the writer. The letter might as well be written to the writer, for the writer, like a diary. She took her sense of her experience through her body and witnessed it.

Then why not keep the letter for herself? Or tear it up? Why send it? Trauma is so intimate. Why share it? Why was that necessary? Burney had been a professional writer for more than thirty years when she had her mastectomy. She might have reread her letter with at least one professional eye. "I resisted all that was resistable." She could evaluate her assertion—her *mot juste.*

She also might imagine she was learning to endure her own thoughts; then, in rereading her letter again, she imagined more than endurance, that stiffening, hardening. She imagined more—survival, transcendence, mastery. The idea of mastery begins a different relationship of writer to the text. It is a relationship that confuses the benefits of composition with the wish to master the past.

The writer might conclude, "There, I wrote it down. I emerged from my paragraphs alive. And yet *another* paragraph might prove I am even more alive than I recently observed." The idea of mastery is often a hasty reaction formed to diminish the too-vivid difficulties of composition, such as violent, invasive memories; resistant ones; rhetorical aggravation; myriad structural and word choices; disturbing fantasies in a tumult with the past. The desire for mastery, coupled with professional pride, could persuade the writer to share what she has made.

"I wrote to my beloved absent sister, and if I send it off to her, she must read it. I know she will read it." But with that hope begins another set of complications. What if the reader is more than an extension or projection of the writer? The reader may be a beloved absent sister, in "reality" and for the purposes of composition, but when the letter moves out of the writer's hand into the world, the reader takes on other roles. Then, for a moment, leave Fanny Burney holding the last page of her letter in the air. She is soothed by her divulgence to Esther. The letter is still in her hand.

> *We hate poetry that has a palpable design upon us.*
> —*John Keats*

After Fanny Burney's letter was published posthumously, a woman choosing to publish her thoughts on breast cancer faced a different task. She could still write to her beloved absent sister and send the letter or not, but when she considered a wider audience, she could not imagine, if she thought about it, that as a subject for composition, this was new. No matter how terrible her fresh wounds, Fanny Burney's letter was always there to throw a long comparative shadow on her chronicles of pain. Burney survived a surgery without anesthesia. What would be the goal of a second, less excruciating version of this narrative, or a third? Would readers compare the sufferings, or the telling of them, on shifting aesthetic grounds, just as the writer made such comparisons, privately?

A defensiveness then works its way into the later writer's work, a defensiveness designed to justify her publication. A woman defends her right to speak; yes, we are back in that familiar scenario. (My mother heard her grandmother say, "A lady's mouth is most attractive closed.") Then a flurry of rhetorical questions follows; or apologies; a self-conscious reaching into history for community; casting about for a significance outside herself; overemphasizing the significance of suffering; until she finds that the most common justifications are *compulsion* and *utility.*

Compulsion: This position surfaces as "I ordinarily would not speak of the breast/the cancer/the medical community/the insurance industry and corporate greed/the multinational carcinogens/the child's deeply disturbed response to my surgery, but X compelled me—" And X is the pain, the cost, the unmanageable emotional response; that is, X is out of the ordinary; mesmerizing, because shocking; and somehow not part of the writer, not assimilated yet. "The horrors that I witnessed/experienced compelled me to speak. I was forced," and then hurdled herself over some implicit modesty. Modesty is the premise. Compulsion, as an argument for writing or publication, is an argument of aberration, perversity. The writer is driven out of herself—made different, larger—and only then will she speak.

Utility: This defense of a woman's public statement is more common. The writer implies that her suffering may have a purpose after all; her pain may serve as one stranger's difficult catharsis. She will be of use to others. It is a Christian paradigm.

In 1972, former child star Shirley Temple Black was the first "celebrity" to "go public" with her mastectomy. She said, "I wanted to help my sisters..." In 1977, First Lady Betty Ford held a press conference before the lump in her breast was removed. Like Black, she wanted to help other women and urged them to examine themselves. Ford said, "I want to help other women..." And she did. Women looked at their breasts in small bathroom mirrors. They touched themselves and learned to touch themselves. They paid for mammograms. (I remember newscasters on the TV in my parents' living room asking each other how many women had Betty Ford and Shirley Temple Black saved when they broke the taboo on breast cancer. Was it hundreds? Thousands? Thousands of women learned from these public figures to "check your breasts.")

Yet when a writer, a poet, a novelist, who has no claim on her country's imagination, nevertheless publishes a poem, a fiction rooted in her suffering, she may insist that the writing is essentially useful. Why? Is she hoping to attach a "higher" purpose to her suffering? Is the "beneficiary" reader a descendent of Fanny Burney's absent sister Esther? To be of use may be a happy thought, a self-enlargement after the amputations of cancer.

Who are the readers of a woman's pain? Who returns to a woman's pain to spend another afternoon going "through it"?

Some readers' response may be similar to the writer's, when she imagined that she mastered her experience by recording it. These readers may feel more alive when they brush up against the edge of written misery. A racing pulse, adrenalin, may follow active reading of someone else's pain. These readers may be imaginatively mobile in their reading, sensing the position of the victim, the palpable wound entered, and moving on, as they like it, to a spectatorial retreat. Is it possible to read a woman's pain without feeling something of her body, her pained body, and is it not a little obscene? Is it sublime? To what extent are these readers conscious of an erotic element in descriptions of a woman's pain? If they are, at all, then these readers could recoil and experience the delicious difference between themselves and the figures in the writer's world. After imagined submergence in the text, they surface, superior, flushed with *Schadenfreude*, more alive.

Other readers may respond much as the traumatized, postwar citizens did in Gunter Grass's *The Tin Drum*. They needed an object to ferret out some semblance of their emotional lives.

These people wanted to talk, to unburden themselves, but they couldn't seem to get started; despite all their efforts, they left the essential unsaid, talked around it. Yet how eager they were to spill their guts, to talk from their hearts, their bowels, their entrails, to forget about their brains just this once . . .

And so the very expensive Onion Cellar opened. Grass's Germans sat on wooden crates covered in burlap, and they waited for their knives and cutting boards and onions. They peeled away each sheer onion skin and then inhaled the onion vapor. "What did the onion juice do? It did what the world and the sorrows of the world could not do: it brought forth a round, human tear. It made them cry. At last they were able to cry again. To cry properly, without restraint . . ."

The reader of a woman's pain may be in search of her own pain, to feel it, assimilate it, master it, imagine she has gone "through it" for the final time. Has she overcome? The reader is reading of another woman's pain and another's, and it is a widening circle of abjection and possible survival, a repetition justified as therapy. Is reading therapeutic if, hour after hour, she is still reading? Compulsion may be disguised as utility. The reader of a woman's pain may be oblivious of her own aggressive desires. One way to approach her own rage is to imagine—or voraciously read of— some other woman's pain. There are many reasons why the market for versions of a woman's pain is so enormous.

(My mother was forty-five when she first had breast cancer. She survived twenty-five years of recurrences: a second breast removed and tumors on scar tissue of earlier surgeries. By the end, she joked with her doctors that her chest wall illustrated the evolution of breast cancer treatment: the radical mastectomy, no longer routine; the infection-riddled skin grafts; the cobalt therapy, now considered carcinogenic; her years of radiation and chemotherapy and electronic beam.)

Fanny Burney's surgery was a success. She lived another thirty years. She had no recurrences. And she continued to support her family—her penniless, aristocratic, and adoring husband and her son—with her novels.

Before her surgery, she sold *Camilla; or, A Picture of Youth* and earned enough money to buy a cottage in the country with some land. "Camilla Cottage," she called it. *The Wanderer; or, Female Difficulties* was her last novel, published in 1814. But the early "sprightliness" was gone. Subsequent novels were mainly commercial projects. For a time, though, she was considered Samuel Richardson's true literary heir. Virginia Woolf called her "the mother of English fiction."

My mother gave me her sleeveless cotton shirts after her mastectomy. I was twelve that summer and hid the shirts, almost out of sight, flattened at the bottom of my drawer. I was afraid that if she saw me in her cool white shirts, she would remember her mastectomy. Years later, when I entered the world, I wore a soft, loose, long-sleeved, transparent blouse. Braless, breasts visible, I was soothed by my display, and not aware of it, not aware that I was not my dear, mutilated mother.

Judith Hall

❦

St. Peregrinus' Cancer

His miracles abbreviated, *Lives of Saints*
        Elaborates his pain:
The famous field he crossed, obliquely, like a crab.
        Silver-pointed crickets
Fanned away, hiding from his dogwood stick,
        His cap on auburn grass.
The clover smelled of local wine, and there
        His vanity could end.

The caption, "Byzantine and Mediterranean,"
        Appeared in my edition
As "Bizarre and sweaty." He was bizarre and sweaty
        Crossing the field in pain.
The parables he hoped the baffled children would
        Recite turned back to babble.

And grass *was not unlike* his doubt, scorched and growing.
        Not silent or silenced,
Nor what in such despair would silence silence—translated
        "He liked to be alone."
An audience today would understand. He went
        The other way; his name
Meant "crossing the field"; going away, one-legged
        In wild licorice.

He sneezed, ruining his pretty suffering,
      The patron saint of cancer.
Once I asked for his crisis, tattooed on my thigh.
      A conversation piece,
Approachable: "Hello. I see by your thigh
      You want to be alone."

Or "Haven't we met? I know your thigh is not unlike
      My own..." A mock-romantic
Brutalism elected with these mutilations.
      And then declare "Cut here,"
To pierce: A gouge for cloisonné; a drowsy blue
      Carves in skin, "*my love.*"
My mother chronicled her cobalt, chemo,
      Then tamoxifen.

Her years of this; her "'*Bravery,*' the doctors said."
      We picked at crab imperials.
I wished for more. I couldn't help it, imagining
      A swoon in cold moiré.
Have and overcome, have and overcome,
      And then I did. I had

The diagnosis; surgery; a souvenir of stitches,
      Pink-stemmed flushes,
Shades of plasma; doubled burgundies and dusky
      Roses; weltered flesh;
The mottled violet and flattened mauve corsages;
      Burnt sienna tissue;
Hardy musk and moss maroon; Madame de Pompadour,
      Ancestor rose! We laughed,

A ladies' lunch, where overarcing hats with velvet
        Clover met; a field
I'd never seen before. The undulating veils
        Of air and grass became
"*You're thin, so thin, so thin, so thin, so thin,*" so then,
        We were alike, at last.

Safiya Henderson-Holmes

❦

"C"-ing in Colors

White

1.

The other.

Ever since being black and female, I've been held in a narrowness of pointing fingers and awkward stares. Ever since my hair's been coarse and nappy, and the dry grayness my mama calls "ash" crept onto my elbow and knees, I knew that whoever touched me would have to walk through the pointed fingers, widen the narrowness, risk it snapping back, and touch me.

Another.

I knew and know difference as air, invisible and familiar, maybe not enough, some days gagging in this skin. some nights breathless

2.

as I stole and hid with my daddy's secret magazines which grew in his closet above his good Sunday clothes. In the magazines were pictures of women whose hair and skin didn't look like mine or mama's. I looked at pictures of their breasts, watched my own rise in their dark quiet softness, slept with those pictures and those women, smiled at my daddy across the dinner table, and blessed my plate with prayers to become the woman of my daddy's magazines. Difference gone from me forever and ever. Amen.

3.

In a stark, white hospital, my black female body between its sheets, sutured and gauzed, pierced with tubing, squares of small plastic bags above and below. I am another "other." The pointed finger submits to "illness," the awkward stare lowers to read statistics. My name's written in a loose-leaf binder and placed in a metal box clipped to the foot of my bed. I am "the

4.

one" near the window.

5.

I'm a sister with three brothers, lived in the Bronx, Soundview pro-jects, seventh floor, 7G. I wanted my own room, my own princess phone and bed, beaded curtains for my window. I wanted to kick my younger brother out, smother his snores, tear his baseball heroes from my walls, fumigate his scent from my closet, put flow-ers and lava lamps in each corner, lay and dare to keep my room just this way.

6.

Bed "B." Is she awake?

7.

I pray for my brothers to come here, stand in the way of this hos-pital bed, bring a gang of snores, crowd the walls with their smells, junk up this narrow closet with their big shoes and pants, make a stink of the night table, air missile the pills and the kidney shaped bowl, shout sport scores, cartwheel for their winners, stomp out their losers. Color these sheets with the girlfriends' lipsticks.

8.

I slept with my younger brother when he was five and I was eight. Before sleeping, we'd make shadow hand puppets on the walls: duck, dog, and rabbit silhouettes, which talked and grazed long after our hands tucked under our sheets. My brother and I slept back to back on our twin bed. Our small, round buns touched slightly. Our elbows, restless wings of rare and clumsy birds, took flight from their sleep every now and then. And every now and then, in the morning, I'd wake and find my brother's head and snores on my chest and I'd hold them there. My brother and I.

9.

Bed "A." Is she awake?

A newcomer is rolled in, an elder woman, white, her arms quietly crossing her chest. Her breasts once full, fuller than my mama's breasts, now kneel in her armpits. Though different, we're dressed in the same thin, pale cloth and colors of this room, like me, her arms weep under the gauze. I watch the invisible and familiar.

An entourage of I.V. poles and plastic tubes, a hum of pumped oxygen, an aria of squeaking wheels, tape, rubber gloves. She's lifted by six hands from stretcher to bed, centered, the blanket unfolding over her stomach. Her rest appears easy. The Demerol bag half full.

I listen to the invisible and familiar:

The beep on the I.V. monitor, a foot rubbing against a crisp sheet, finger tremors against the railing, the turning of a breath.

And then I hear her snore. Loud and long. Like a member of my family. Like my brother.

10.

Moving on to my chest.

Pink

1.

dream:

Night, dark gray sky, no moon, no stars. I'm running, breathless, naked, a large bouquet of roses in both hands. I don't feel the thorns, but I see them piercing my skin. Red petals dropping, wet grass under my feet, mud, tiny rocks, sticks. I slip, fall, mud and rose petals on my hands and knees. I stand, run again, holding the roses tightly. A wind is chasing me. I run faster. More red petals falling into wings.

2.

Awake:

In my hospital room, on a small shelf fastened to the wall in front of my hospital bed, is a garden: roses in a white vase, yellow tulips in a glass pitcher, daisies in a yellow paper cup, an aloe plant in a red pot, a philodendron in a blue pot, mums and tiger lilies in a pink vase. A toy bee hovering from a card.

3.

A nurse wearing perfume and red lipstick touches me. Her hand a smooth pink cup. She holds my chin as my mother did when I was a little girl, and my menstrual cramps were too painful to be only a female thing. "I'm the I.V. nurse," she says, "I have to draw some blood." My chin crumbles in her hand.

4.

My veins hide and whenever found roll into the pockets of my flesh and hide again. The perfume and lipstick become hunters, each with a tiny, silver spear. "Think of your beautiful flowers and that bee," the nurse says. My vein leaps. My skin stings. No blood. No mercy. The perfume and lipstick disguise themselves with patience.

5.

dream:

The virgin is rarely told about pain and never is the flower, both are fragrant and open, placed in a soft bed. When the gatherers of honey appear, the virgin and the flower sense something other than delight in the buzz and the hum, in the push and suck, but they also sense that life may depend on this. Below bone, below corolla, the virgin and the flower know how sweetness is made, how sweetness survives.

6.

The tulips are from Anna, she's had two miscarriages in one year, her one child, a daughter, is deaf and takes ballet classes after school. To pay for ballet, Anna does magic tricks at children's parties. She swallows fire. The aloe plant's from Bob. His wife of twenty-some-odd years died of lung cancer a month ago. He says aloes are good healers. He has a shot of aloe juice and tequila every day. The mums and tiger lilies are Sarah's, she's always saying how good she grows flowers and husbands, then cuts them at the root and gives them to friends. She has a very large and lush garden and many friends. The roses are from Judy, a pretty cocobrown woman with a moonblue left eye. The philodendron is Pete's, Judy's friend. Sometimes he worries about his whiteness next to Judy's blackness. I tell him to worry about her moonblue eye. The daisies and card with the bee were here when I arrived.

7.

A vein surrenders, thread thin in my left hand. The lipstick smiles. I watch my blood empty into two small plastic vials. The spears are tossed. The smooth pink cup holds my chin again, "Now, which flower were you?"

8.

dream:

Rose petals falling into wings. I'm running, the wind lifting my hair and skin, my skin covering the sky. A full moon rising on my face.

9.

Tomorrow I'm sure my mother will bring me peonies.

Annette Williams Jaffee

❧

The Good Mother

The good mother often dies at the beginning of the story.
—*Marina Warner,* From the Beast to the Blonde

1. Myths

THE YEAR MY MOTHER STARTED TO DIE I WAS thirteen. My mother was dying in the front bedroom but I was on the porch reading novels and eating those tart green grapes that later I would not eat because of Chavez and injustice. It was a small square brick porch, jutting off one side of the front of the house. Next to it was a Rose of Sharon bush that in the summer gave out large crepey blossoms with hard bristly stamens. In the back of the house was a full lilac bush and sometimes, in the spring, I would push out the screen of the dormer window of my bedroom and climb onto the roof and bury my face in the heavy scent. Sometimes I would sit on the roof and smoke forbidden cigarettes.

My mother was fiercely proud of those two bushes and of our house, she was mad for hope and beauty. They meant that all was not squalor or in vain and that she had her rightful place in the world. It was an ordinary brick bungalow on an ordinary city street, but it was all she would have in the whole world now.

The porch and the wide concrete steps that led to it, and the flowering bushes were all I remembered about the house for a long time because I was not there. I was in Wessex as Tess tells the story of her betrayal to Angel Clare and on the train when Sister Carrie meets Drouet, and in Rouen with Emma Bovary as the cab wildly circled the city, the window curtains pulled tight, Leon's shouted excited instructions: to drive!

Years later, when I went places and rode in the back seats of taxis and woke in the night in high foreign beds in cities not entirely familiar to me, I could be the girl on the porch, but not for a long time. I needed the relief of distance before I could have my childhood and before I could remember my mother's suffering; I was that terrified of not escaping.

My mother's illness had been diagnosed that summer: cancer of the breast, although it was not what I was told. When I think of how I was told, I see a Greek chorus of talking heads: bright colored carnival heads, the bobbing heads of arcade games, nodding velour dogs on the flat back platforms of cars in the fifties, huge elastic mouths moving, loose tongues flapping, whispering nonsense syllables, an occasional recognizable word escaping. The word I remember was *arthritis*. Certainly that made some sense as my mother was in a wheelchair when I went to visit her in the hospital. (This visit was supposed to be reassuring.) A friend at school gave me the real word. "Oh, Annette," she said, "I'm sorry your mother has cancer." I hated that girl from then on, hated her for telling the truth.

First her breast was removed. Treatment, rudimentary then, involved shots of male hormones that caused my mother to grow a thick mustache and a rough dark beard. Her female organs were scooped out; radiation caused burning of the skin around her ravaged chest and back. No one in my family spoke of my mother's condition to me again, nor was it given another name. I could have pointed to things: the ragged scars glimpsed from a casually closed robe, the coarse facial hair only partly removed by the smelly depilatory, the terrible rubber breast form poking out of a half-open drawer, but I did not. The mythology surrounding my mother's sickness and the continued observance of that mythology seemed central to her survival.

When my mother was not sleeping, she read. Sometimes I was called from the porch. I don't remember what my mother talked about then; perhaps she asked what I was reading. I do remember my replies were curt, impatient, surly. Sometimes she needed water to take her medication. Sometimes she had to be helped to the toilet. A maid came everyday now, a tall black woman who rode the el all the way across Chicago, from the south side to the north and back, in a pair of carpet slippers and a man's raincoat.

At five the doctor arrived with his glasses and his worn square bag to give my mother a shot for pain. He had instructed me to boil water in a small tin saucepan, to sterilize the hypodermic needle. I left the room quickly then, but not before I heard their voices and my mother's grateful gasp.

2. Heroines

Chapter One: In which we meet our headstrong heroine and learn the details of her dangerous plan.

These words appear in a pretentious leather-bound notebook in November 1981, the day before I was about to undergo prophylactic bilateral mastectomies, a surgical procedure I usually described—depending on my audience—as slicing off my breasts.

As casual as I liked to sound, it was the final step in a highly calculated course I had been on most of my life. When I was ten, my grandmother died of breast cancer. My mother died when I was sixteen; she was forty-one. I didn't know if it was part of a European inheritance or something entirely New World, but it belonged to me, as surely as their thick hair and big hips, small hands and feet, and the Haviland soup bowls. I was thirty-six, the mother of two early adolescent children; my first novel had been published that spring; but like some peasant in a medieval passion play, death was the keystone of my life.

The journey to save my own life was begun in earnest the week after my father's death. I was thirty-one and an orphan, and my father's death freed me to own my mother's death. The mythology of her illness had been kept intact except for oblique references and asides that allowed him to know that I knew.

My father used to get slightly weepy if we were alone (my stepmother allowed no such lapses on her watch), and he would take my hand and ask if I ever thought about my mother. I grabbed my hand back when I was younger and let him hold it as I grew older, but mainly I'd say yes, and then he'd launch into the catechism. Did I check my breasts? Yes. Do you remember to tell the doctors how old Mommy was when she died? Yes. And that Grandma died from it, too? Yes. And you remember to tell them about the radiation treatments?

Yes. I had been born with a hemangioma, a bloody cyst on my left breast. Radiation, one of the precious legacies of the Second World War, was being used to treat this and similar birthmarks; doctors were now finding malignancies in people who had undergone these treatments as children. I had received eight separate doses of radiation to that breast in the first year of my life.

Now I was the keeper of my own breasts and the first thing I did was make an appointment with a plastic surgeon who was a proponent of a surgical procedure called subcutaneous mastectomies. In this, the outer layer of breast skin was lifted, as much breast tissue as possible was removed and then replaced immediately with silicone implants. Voilà! "Subcutaneous Mastectomies: An Operation in Search of Patients" was the title of a scholarly article this doctor had written. I arrived in his office wearing the black dress I had worn to my father's funeral the week before, so tense that he had to pass me a Valium before he could examine me.

But he sent me to the right place, a breast cancer specialist in New York, a tiny elderly gentleman with a thin silver mustache, a toupée, and the rosette of the Knights of Malta nestled into the buttonhole of his white coat. I soon became one of the youngest of the supplicants, squeezed into a waiting room full of the faithful, surrounded by the floor-to-ceiling framed evidence of our hero's accomplishments and supporters. Somewhere in this maze of pious personalities was a small engraving of Saint Agatha, patron saint of breast diseases, her naked outstretched arms offering her own breasts like bonbons on a silver platter. For the first time since my mother's diagnosis I felt safe: safe with my secrets, my fears. I will offer my breasts and save my own stupid life.

3 . Scavengers

My mother loved pistachio nuts. I can see her biting through the tiny slit, and her fingers and front teeth and lips turning a brazen red from the dye they used. She loved pomegranates, too, although I have never learned to eat them. I remember her leaning over the sink or a large linen napkin sucking and spitting out the seeds. I wonder if she mentioned the myth of Demeter; it was her way of doing things, connecting the lives of the ancient gods with our own small lives for me. She loved popcorn, too, buttered, salted popcorn—chewing your cud, my father used to say, laughing when he saw her dip into a box of it at the movies.

And she loved pumpkin seeds. On Halloween, she and I carefully scooped them out before we carved a huge pumpkin from the supermarket on an old kitchen table brought out to the porch for this purpose. It was cold by then and I warmed my hands in the front of her sweater or she would place them on her warm cheeks or blow onto them, almost putting them in her mouth. We separated the plump white seeds from the orangey pulp and dried them on newspapers, and the next day, when I went to school as Cinderella or Little Red Riding Hood, she roasted them in the oven on baking sheets blackened with use and covered them with coarse salt. I never got the hang of eating those, either; it didn't seem worth it, that narrow splinter of tenderness. Usually, I ate the whole thing, getting it caught in my throat and giving up in a flurry of dramatic choking.

My mother loved the bony parts of chicken, too: the wings, feet, neck; she would scoop marrow from the meat bones that came from a barley soup. My mother was a scavenger, I realized years later; she loved the sweet surprise at the end of the struggle, she loved the bony gristly challenge of it.

4 . Theatrical Events

Early in 1981, a small lump no one is worried about is biopsied, just to see. There are pre-cancerous changes in the cells and we move the activity up a notch. I enter a time of winter darkness, taxis whisking me and my slides around New York into the Persian-rug-spread waiting rooms of Park Avenue brownstones and up and down the glass and marble corridors of Memorial Sloan-Kettering Hospital. The doctors agree: why not? It becomes obvious that they have no real answers for this: they cannot cure, they can merely catch it in time. A week before the surgery, as I am trying to give my own blood (too late) at the hospital where I will have the surgery, I suddenly panic. I cannot do this. I am too young, I am wearing blue jeans, I have a Bloomingdale's charge card.

The night before the surgery, having finally fallen asleep into a black dreamless drugged sleep, I awaken to see a large, distinguished, completely bald man dressed in evening clothes seated by my bedside. For one minute I think I have died and God is dressed in black tie, as I had always hoped He would be. It is the anesthesiologist paying his required call. He has been to the opera: *Tosca*.

My mother's brother, in New York on business, visits me the day after surgery. I am still so foggy all I remember is a dimly lit stage set, a misty New York autumn afternoon, a glimpse of the Chrysler Building through a window. He and I and my I.V. take a slow stroll up and down the hall. He tells the nurses I am his baby, that he used to push me in my carriage in Texas where I was born at the end of the war; he tells them to take care of me. I wave weakly. Is he remembering other hospital visits: his mother, my mother? This seems an odd rite of passage in a family.

The third day the lady from the American Cancer Society visits with her toys: a short rope, a rubber ball, cotton pads to stuff in my bra. I am bright and perky, I am cooperative and funny, I am the good girl student. I sit cross-legged on my bed, my dirty hair pulled into a ponytail, in rapt attention, nodding pleasantly at everything. I am utterly stupid, of course; an hour after she leaves, I realize I am the mastectomy patient she was talking about.

Home from the hospital, my thirteen-year-old son fixes me with a careful gaze. "You look different," he says.

"Yeah?" There's no pretending here. I've told both my children what's up, no mumbo jumbo this time around.

"Did you cut your hair?"

"No. I told you I…"

"That's it, you look shorter," he decides and quickly exits stage right.

The metaphor of theater is not completely wrong: such events open one to fantasy, to make-believe, to bullshit. For the next three months before I can begin reconstruction, I wear large men's Brooks Brothers shirts in pink and yellow, I buy some fantastic silk and lace camisoles. I wear a long strand of pearls day and night. I am not going to fake breasts. The plastic surgeon, an expert in fantasy, tells me he has had models in his office who are flatter-chested than I.

In February, I have the implants. This time it hurts; I am not the good girl patient. They carve into the wall of my chest to put the silicone blobs under muscle. There is an accumulation of blood on one side that needs to be painfully aspirated twice a week, and for a month I live and breathe, sleep, and eat in a bone corset, like one of the women in *The Story of O*.

In May, they make nipples from skin cut from my groin. The incisions in the groin are sewn loosely—so you can walk, the surgeon explains casually, and the wounds weep; they require the frequent application of saline compresses. I make the solution myself.

The following year the outer rims of the implants pop and I have to replace them. This time they use solid gel that hardens and feels heavier. I have had four surgical procedures in less than eighteen months, but I'm still cracking jokes. Just like me, I say, to spend months and thousands of dollars to replace something I already had.

Of course, they're not really breasts. They remind me of a comment made by a Swedish friend about American coffee. It's a hot brown beverage, all right, he said, but it's not coffee. Well, there are two round things sticking out, but they're not breasts.

5. Inheritance

My daughter is twenty-seven. She has just moved to a new apartment and I am engaged in the ancient exchange ritual of helping her set up house and cleaning out my garage at the same time. We pull out the Haviland creamed-soup bowls and saucers that are the end of my grandmother's china.

She shrugs; there are three bowls left. "I have plenty of bowls, Mom."

I read everything I can about genetic testing, although I don't need science to determine the need: my mother, my grandmother, her younger sister, the eldest daughter of the older sister, and one of this daughter's daughters. These are the ones I know about.

My daughter makes plans for a life in international trade, she talks about getting a dog, raising children, saving developing nations. She speaks several languages, flies to exotic places on business. At her age I had two small children and one goal: I wanted to outlive my mother. Being the perfect mother was simple. I wanted to live long enough to watch them grow up. Doctors told me to have my children young, close together, and to breast feed. My entire youth became sublimated to this. But then I decided to trick death, elude it, preempt it. Of course, by doing this I have to admit I have outdone my mother, that she wasn't clever enough to do it for me, that in some basic way, I am a better mother than my mother was. It is hard to give up the idea of the perfection of a dead mother.

What does my daughter know of this? The habit of not talking is strong. When Betsy turned twenty-one, I dragged her to a breast cancer clinic. They taught her a certain number of things about checking herself, but they didn't seem alarmed by her family history and she doesn't have the reels of horror movies of my childhood. After all, I made sure she didn't.

I have been sorting through the one carton that now contains not only my life and my children's childhoods but both my parents' lives. There was more, of course—diplomas and dance bids, military discharges, yellowing newspaper headlines, but it was not of much interest to me and so over the years it succumbed to the natural disasters of time and neglect and was tossed out.

Mice have gotten into this box over the long winter. It is in the attic of a very old house and soon we will all be reduced to this, we will have become a mound of mauled and toothed scraps, anyway. My mother has been dead for thirty-five years; there is not much left of her, I am sure, in a grave I have not seen since we buried my father next to her twenty years ago. Sometimes I think death gave me this vocation, this need to conjure up lives with so little real information. When my grandmother was dying, I was ten and was busily writing a book about her imagined childhood. The only thing I knew about her was that she had been born in Meriden, Connecticut, not a real place to me, only a name. No one told me she was dying, either, no one told me why, but somehow I thought the book might keep her alive. I was wrong, and I was right; words and memory are all I have of so many people I loved as a child.

It has taken me thirty-five years to put out a photograph of my mother next to the desk where I write. It is a tinted copy of a photograph my father carried all his life, my mother as a sixteen-year-old college freshman, the year my father met her, the first day of classes in a survey course of Western Civilization. She was sitting in the front row, a flat pump dangling from her toes until it dropped into my father's hand. For their first date they went to see the newly released movie *Snow White and the Seven Dwarfs*. They ate ice cream at Henrici's in cold, silver, footed cups. The details of their streetcar romance were as familiar to me as the ones in the fairy tales I loved. Except I had to witness the ever-after. Dreamy, dreamy, those were my parents, from fairy tales to Chekhov, where the grown-ups floated through empty rooms, listening to the little night music playing in their heads, their noses in books.

From my mother's college notebooks:

> *Sons and Lovers*—primarily the story of a mother fixation.
> Leo Tolstoy—the motive which dominates his novels is the portrayal of characters through the mighty passions of men and women. In real life.
> *Of Mice and Men*—underlying theme: danger of dreaming.

6. The Good Mother

The last time I saw my mother, an aunt and I had been shopping downtown and we stopped at the hospital. My father took my aunt for a walk down the hall and I sat, impatient, scraping my feet along the floor, slouched in the chair next to my mother's hospital bed. I barely answered some questions: what I ate for lunch, what I bought. Bored, I ran out to the water fountain for a drink and saw my father and my aunt. His arm was around her and she was weeping onto his shoulder. In a second I knew. I ran back to my mother's bed and threw my arms around her. I began to sob. "Oh, please, Mommy, please, promise me you won't die," I begged her as I wept. She held me very tight and promised she wouldn't die.

I never saw my mother again. A week later she died in that hospital bed in the middle of the night. I heard the phone ring and I went downstairs. My father and his sister were sitting together at the kitchen table. We drank tea with a little whiskey poured into it. None of us cried, and they talked about people and places from long ago, from a time that did not belong to me or my mother but before my father had ever met my mother.

I still see her everywhere. I see her standing in the kitchen in a pink shirtwaist dress, a grosgrain ribbon tied in her neat dark hair, waiting to hear about my school day. I see her sitting on the stairs that led upstairs, talking on the telephone to one of my aunts or one of her college friends—the V.D. Sisters, they called themselves, a group of recent girl graduates, social workers unprepared but game to handle the cases with venereal diseases they were assigned. I remember her face lighting up with joy as she described Maria Tallchief's *Firebird.*

Even in the worst of times, the ballet was our secret language. I have studio portraits of my mother at nine, *en pointe,* her elaborate headdress like a fringed lampshade. Her copy of Romola's *Life of Nijinsky* sits on my shelf. I wish I had the ballerina pins with pink and blue stone tutus that danced across the lapel of a gray wool suit. I see her sitting on the bench in the changing room, knitting and chatting with the other mothers as I took my ballet classes every Saturday for years and years.

For months after my mother's death, her magazines continued to come: *Ladies Home Journal* and *McCall's* and I would, in my sixteen-year-old way, both reject them and hungrily read about being a mother, a housewife, a cook and hostess. I knew she was buried in her gray-blue silk dress because I saw that it was missing from her closet the morning after her death when I went into her bedroom to snoop around, the way I always did.

My mother's blue-rimmed eyeglasses were folded on her dresser tray; my father had brought them home from the hospital after he had made the arrangements. I remember thinking how nearsighted she was and I worried about how she could get along without her glasses.

Eve Kosofsky Sedgwick

❧

White Glasses

*(Originally presented at a conference at the City University of New
York's Center for Lesbian and Gay Studies, May 9, 1991)*

> Today as you passed a dark-skinned
> man younger than you
> his eyes plucked yours (Indian? West Indian?),
> set you to wondering what he
> saw: a close-cropped man
> with briefcase, white rolled
> shorts, white glasses,
>
> a lope on tiptoes, a
> scowl, blue eyes behind the frames,
> licking a cone of ice cream...[1]

1.

THE FIRST TIME I MET MICHAEL LYNCH, I THOUGHT
his white-framed glasses were the coolest thing I had ever seen. It
was at the Modern Language Association Convention, in New
York, in 1986. My first thought was, "Within two months, every
gay man in New York is going to be wearing white glasses." My
second thought: "Within a year, every fashion-conscious person in
the United States is going to be wearing white glasses." My instant
resolve: "I want to wear white glasses first.

When I first met Michael Lynch in December of 1986, it was
at an informal coffee-shop breakfast meeting to discuss the possibility of putting out an annual volume of essays in gay and lesbian studies. It wasn't a big breakfast—eight or nine people in a
coffee shop—but there was room, at that early though star-
tlingly recent moment in the institutionalization of gay/lesbian

studies for almost everyone who had actually published a book in the field, plus a few, like Michael, who hadn't yet. The project was Michael's project because throughout the history of gay studies, of gay activism since Stonewall, Michael has been somebody who has catalyzed, crystallized, fecundated projects, institutions, and communities wherever he has been—wherever geographically, wherever institutionally, wherever in identity and experience.

The day I first met Michael Lynch in New York was the day that, in Toronto, the complicated, arbitrary diagnostic process around AIDS finally caught up with Michael's ex-lover, housemate, best-loved friend, a medical researcher, Bill Lewis, who was to die suddenly the next fall. I heard Michael telling friends around MLA about Bill's diagnosis; I saw the traces of Bill's diagnosis in the amazing dignity and openness with which Michael introduced and chaired a panel I had organized (I, who didn't in 1986 personally know anyone with AIDS) on AIDS and homophobic discourse; the Michael I met and fell in love with was, to some degree I could never estimate, a Michael made different on the same day by the suddenly more graphic proximity of intimate loss—perhaps also by the availability of comfort from friends, and even by the public performance under the MLA's weirdly legitimating and routinizing aegis of an AIDS-activist discourse entirely new to that particular theater. Michael's availability to be identified with and loved, in my instant, fetishistic crystallization of him through those white glasses, must have had everything to do with my witness of this moment. At the same time I have always felt, since then, that the important ways in which I *haven't* gotten to know Michael fully are somehow coextensive with my never having known Bill. The same loss, the same history of struggle and subtraction made Michael available to my identification and love, opaque to my knowledge.

And the I who met Michael and fell in love with his white glasses? It was nobody simpler than the handsome and complicated poet and scholar I met in him; it was a queer but long-married young woman whose erotic and intellectual life were fiercely transitive, shaped by a thirst for knowledges and identifications that might cross the barriers of what seemed my identity. It was also someone who had it at heart to make decisive interventions on two scenes of identity that were supposed not to have to do with each other: the scene of feminism, where I "identified" and which I knew well; and the scene of gay men's bonding, community, thought, and politics, a potent and numinous scene which at the experiential level was at that time almost totally unknown to me.

2.

When I decided to write "White Glasses" for a conference on lesbian and gay studies, I thought it was going to be an obituary for Michael Lynch. The best thing about writing it is that it isn't— it's an act of homage to a living friend—but someday it will be. I thought I would have to do the speaking of it, and probably the thinking and writing for it, after Michael's death of AIDS-related infection. Which seemed imminent. After months of grogginess, discontinuous attention, extreme weakness, futile attempts to regain weight and alertness, Michael had decided it was time to die: time to end the assaultive doses of antibiotics, to stop stuffing himself with food he didn't want, to take the decision about his fate back into the autonomous hands where it belonged. In making the decision to let himself die, refusing food and all but palliative care, Michael was supported by amazing resources of affection, information, and the most mundane personal care from the communities he himself created, co-created, and fostered in Toronto. Old and new friends, from *The Body Politic*, from AIDS Action Now!, and from the Canadian Center for Gay and Lesbian Studies—the last of these a new organization Michael had founded in response to Bill Lewis's death—organized a care team for Michael on what I think is an unprecedented model and scale:

twenty-four-hour-a-day attendance by a weekly rota of thirty or so friends, organized through Sunday meetings (often with a nurse), instructed and kept scrupulous track of through a massive log book.... Empowerment to decide, permission to die, the knowledge and tending necessary to do so on his own terms—these turned out to have been not only among the many gifts from the people who love Michael but also a part of Michael's legacy to himself from two decades of activism, writing, and what can only be called the work of community.

3.

It took me a year and a half of peering in the window of every optician in New York, northern California, and Massachusetts to find glasses that I thought looked like Michael's. When I got them I felt fashion perfect—I felt like Michael—even though, in the intervening time, the predicted fashion craze of white glasses had entirely failed to materialize. When I got the glasses I also learned from watching, through them, the faces of other people looking at me, that although to me the glasses meant (mean) nothing but Michael, to others—even to people who know Michael—the glasses don't.

One thing I learned from this is that the white of the glasses means differently for a woman, for a man. The white of the glasses is two things, after all. White is a color—it is a pastel. White the pastel sinks banally and invisibly into the camouflage of femininity, on a woman, a white woman. In a place where it doesn't belong, on Michael, that same pastel remains a flaming signifier.

White is also, however, at the same time no color, the color of color's own subtraction and absence. At once the white-flaring acid of dissolution, the acid's crystalline residue and its voided trail; in many cultures white is the color of mourning. On women of all colors white refers, again banally, to virginity (to virginity as absence or to the absence of virginity) and the flirta-

tions of the veil—to the ways in which our gender tries to construct us heterosexually as absence and as the dissimulating
denial of it, and tries also to inscribe in us, as a standard of our
own and other people's value, the zero-degree no-color of (not
the skin of Europeans themselves but) the abstractive ideology of
European domination. A white woman wearing white: the ruly
ordinariness of this sight makes invisible the corrosive aggression
that white also is: as the blaze of mourning, the opacity of loss,
the opacity loss installs within ourselves and our vision, the
unreconciled and irreconcilably incendiary energies streaming
through that subtractive gap, that ragged scar of meaning,
regard, address.

4.

When I decided to write "White Glasses" four months ago I
thought my friend Michael Lynch was dying and I thought I was
healthy. Unreflecting, I formed my identity as the prospective
writer of this piece around the obituary presumption that my own
frame for speaking, the margin of my survival and exemption, was
the clearest thing in the world. In fact it was totally opaque:
Michael didn't die; I wasn't healthy: within the space of a couple of
weeks, we were dealing with a breathtaking revival of Michael's
energy, alertness, appetite—also with my unexpected diagnosis
with a breast cancer already metastasized to several lymph nodes.
So I got everything wrong. I thought I knew back then that assign-
ing myself this task in advance, for this conference whose audience
I knew would include many of Michael's friends, people who have
known him much longer and better than I, as well as people who
might never have heard of him and others who know him only as
a defining figure in the story of gay studies—I thought it was a
good way to deal prospectively and perhaps lucidly with a process
of shock and mourning about Michael's loss that had, indeed,
already become turbidly disruptive in my life to a degree I found I
couldn't share more directly with Michael. Memorials, dedications:

places where you say as if to someone else the things you can't say to the people you love. I thought I would have to—I thought I could—address this to you instead of to Michael; and now I can do both. The I who does both is also a different one with new fears and temporalities, a newly sharpened appreciation of the love of friends and comrades, new experience of amputation and prosthesis, new knowledge, expectations, angers, luxuries, and dependencies. Now shock and mourning gaze in both directions through the obituary frame; and much more than shock and mourning; it is exciting that Michael is alive and full of beans today, sick as he is; I think it is exciting to both of us that I am; and in many ways it is full of stimulation and interest, even, to be ill and writing.

5.

Now, I know I don't "look much like" Michael Lynch, even in my white glasses. Nobody knows more fully, more fatalistically than a fat woman how unbridgeable the gap is between the self we see and the self as whom we are seen; no one, perhaps, has more practice at straining and straining to span the binocular view between; and no one can appreciate more fervently the act of magical faith by which it may be possible, at last, to assert and believe, against every social possibility, that the self we see can be made visible as if through our own eyes to the people who see us. The stubborn magical defiance I have learned (I *sometimes* feel I have succeeded in learning) in forging a habitable identity as a fat woman is also what has enabled the series of uncanny effects around these white glasses; uncanny effects that have been so formative of my—shall I call it my identification? Dare I, after this half decade, call it with all a fat *woman's* defiance, my identity?— as a gay man.

Uncanny effects: effects as of the frame; as of the mask: effects of focal length.

When I am with Michael, often suddenly it will be as if we were fused together at a distance of half an inch from the eye.

Or I will feel as if someone who looked at us might be blinded by the white stigma of our glasses. It sometimes amazes me that anyone can tell us apart.

So often I feel that I see with Michael's eyes—not because we are the same, but because the same prosthetic device attaches to, extends, and corrects the faulty limb of our vision.

It is as if we were both the man in the iron mask; different men in the same iron mask.

When I am in bed with Michael, our white glasses line up neatly on the night table and I always fantasize that I may walk away wearing the wrong ones.

I mention my obsessive imagery to a friend of Michael's, who says, "That's right, I did notice that you and Michael both wear those patio-furniture glasses."

6.

"My identity," along with Michael, "as a gay man," I say. Yet our most durable points of mutual reference are lesbian. My favorite picture of Michael was taken in Willa Cather's bed. We are both obsessed with Emily Dickinson. Tokens, readings, pilgrimages, impersonations around Cather, Dickinson, and our other lesbian ego-ideals shape and punctuate our history. The first thing Michael did after my diagnosis in February was to bundle into the mail to me a blanket that has often comforted me at his house—a blanket whose meaning to him is its association with the schoolteacher aunt whose bed he used to lie in in childhood, sandwiched in the crack between her and her lifelong companion, wondering whether (after all, he was adopted) it might not be this Boston marriage whose offspring he somehow really, naturally was.

If what is at work here is an identification that falls across gender, it falls no less across sexualities, across "perversions." And across the ontological crack between the living and the dead.

7.

Judith Butler in *Gender Trouble:* "Lacan...remarks that 'the function of the mask...dominates the identifications through which refusals of love are resolved'.... In a characteristic gliding over pronominal locations, Lacan fails to make clear who refuses whom. As readers, we are meant, however, to understand that this free-floating 'refusal' is linked in a significant way to the mask. If every refusal is, finally, a loyalty to some other bond in the present or the past, refusal is simultaneously preservation as well. The mask thus conceals this loss, but preserves (and negates) this loss through its concealment. The mask has a double function which is the double function of melancholy. The mask is taken on through the process of incorporation which is a way of inscribing and then wearing a melancholic identification in and on the body; in effect, it is the signification of the boy in the mold of the Other who has [been] refused. Dominated through appropriation, every refusal fails, and the refuser becomes part of the very identity of the refused, indeed, becomes the psychic refuse of the refused."[2]

Michael Moon on Judith Butler: "I am arguing on behalf of sex-radical groups dealing with AIDS for the desirability, indeed, the necessity... of allowing our sex radicalism to pervade our mourning practices to a degree that we have to this point only begun to explore. I believe Butler's analysis of the melancholia of gender has important implications for this possibility.... 'Properly' gendered persons, according to Butler's rereading of Freud, are compelled to deny (first to themselves) that they ever felt desire 'inappropriate' to their supposed desire, and are not permitted to grieve over the loss of this 'other desire.' I want to supplement this perception by arguing that 'melancholy,' homo or hetero, is not just about the disavowal and lack of grieving for '*the* other' desire; there are '*many* other' desires—the entire range of 'perversions'—which many people feel compelled to deny and to omit grieving the loss of.... We want to conduct our mourning and grieving in the image of, and as an indispensable part of, this task of collectively and solitarily exploring 'perverse' or stigmatized desire." [3]

8.

From a letter to my little brother in the summer of 1987:

"If you leafed through the enclosed snapshots before getting to the prose, you'll have inferred from the unusual prevalence of *white enameled glasses* that we had—last weekend—a lovingly anticipated visit from my Toronto friend Michael, along with his 16-year-old son, Stefan. The visit, very eventless on the surface, probably nice in many ways that will be palpable in retrospect, seems to be leaving me with a heavy after-turbulence of feeling inadequate and even *bad,* as well as impotent, awful, and the other more usual affectionate things.

"I realized as soon as they left Sunday that I had had, in advance, a quite specific fantasy about their visit. This went back to the time three years ago, when our friend Jeff was in the hospital in NYC with the sudden crisis of an autoimmune disease. As we understood it, if he could have made it through that crisis, the disease could probably have been managed and he would have been okay. The whole week or so he was in the hospital before he died, I focused all my energies on the mental image of the time in the coming summer when he, his wife, and his about-to-be-born kid would come up to spend a slow, sunny, maybe impossible weekend lying about on the lawn with us in Amherst—which was going to be the sign that he was fine and everything was fine. Of course, this never happened, but I think I must have kept the fantasy in storage: the feeling that if Michael would only bring Stefan here for a summer weekend and if I could only manage to provide exactly the right background of *dolce far niente*, then nothing could really fail to be (and Michael could not really fail to be) *just fine.*

"In fact, I think the pressure of this not quite recognized fantasy probably made it harder for any of us to relax or connect properly this weekend. But it didn't require that to make a problem, either, probably; the plainest fact seemed to be that Michael, while he tried with his usual sweetness to sparkle and connect, was weak and exhausted, and probably the thing he wanted most—I certainly would have—was to be in his own bed in his own house. The evening they got here he talked about being able to just rest and decompress. But that night he had an upsetting dream. He had to get a lot of dead bodies out of drawers in an office in a high-rise building, put them into coffins, and get them down the elevators and onto the street, where they were going to be carried as part of a funeral-cum-AIDS activist demonstration. But it was Halloween, and the elevators were already full of masked and costumed people; throughout the building was the grim, drunken atmosphere of office parties. Then next day we did the tour of Emily Dickinson's house, which I think he found chillingly alienating and weird (I just registered it as normally alienating and weird, but then I'm used to Amherst). Then, because we wanted to look at a video he'd brought, a CBC special, "AIDS and the Arts," in which he figures as the Poet, we went to TV rental/repair place in the center of town that was unmistakably something from the twilight zone: a dark burrow, on a second floor that had no intelligible spatial relation to the ordinary blocks of Amherst that supposedly surrounded it, stuffed with hundreds and hundreds of old dead TVs, and inhabited by two guys who, though young, appeared not to have stepped out of the place in fifty years. Michael almost fainted while we were there, and, though he'd slept till noon, slept again for most of the rest of the afternoon. Then he conked out almost immediately after dinner.... When they finally left, it felt utterly bitter to let them out of sight or to stop hugging him, maybe because it was only physical touch that ever seemed, all weekend, to burn (Michael feels very hot) through the static of concern, distraction, (his) unpredictable fragility, (my) misplaced bustling, distance (whose?)....

"Sentimentality aside, if it ever can be, I've had a hard time processing all this. I have some obvious, even vengefully moralistic things I can tell myself about it (i.e., that things are not fine and not going to be, and in ways that have only minimally to do with any pressure of one's own feelings), but those don't at all answer to the ways in which one does, or may, nonetheless connect—or with the bitterness of not doing so."

9.

Last weekend, visiting Toronto, I had a few minutes to look through the log book kept by Michael's care team. I leafed back to February, to the time of my diagnosis and mastectomy, and was amazed to find that one caregiver's shift after another had been marked by the restlessness, exhaustion, and pain of Michael's anxiety about what was going on with me in Durham. Of course it didn't surprise me that he was worried about me or compassionated with me during such a difficult passage. But what I had felt I was experiencing from him at the time—remember that these were the same weeks when Michael was supposed to die, but instead got stronger and stronger—was the tremendous plenitude of the energies he somehow had available to inject into me. The friend who had been, only weeks before, so flickering and disconnected that I worried that it was torturing him to make him talk on the phone, now was at my ear daily with hours of the lore, the solicitude, the ground-level truthtelling and demand for truthtelling that I simply had to have. I also felt miraculously revitalized by the joy of having a real Michael, not the dry-mouthed struggling shade of him, there again to communicate with. I didn't know where these energies came from in Michael—I thought they were produced as if magically by my need of them; to some extent I still think they were—but I see now that they were also carved directly out of Michael's substance, his rest, and his peace of mind.

But also a lot of what I needed so unexpectedly to learn from Michael I had already had opportunities to learn. So much about how to be sick—how to occupy most truthfully and powerfully, and at the same time constantly to question and deconstruct, the sick role, the identity of the "person living with life-threatening disease"—had long been embodied in him, and performed by him, in ways which many of us, sick and well, have had reason to appreciate keenly. These are skills that could not have evolved outside the context of liberatory identity politics and AIDS activism, but their flavor is also all Michael's own.[4] I have sometimes condensed them to myself in the unbearably double-edged performative injunction, "Out, out—." As if the horrifying fragility of a life's brief flame could somehow be braced and welded, in the forge of the signifier, as if orthopedically to the galvanizing coming-out imperative of visibility, defiance, solidarity, and self-assertion. From Michael I also seem always to hear the injunction—not the opposite of "Out, out" but somehow a part of it—"Include, include": to entrust as many people as one possibly can with one's actual body and its needs, one's stories about its fate, one's dreams, and one's sources of information or hypothesis about disease, cure, consolation, denial, and the state or institutional violence that are also invested in one's illness. It's as though there were transformative political work to be done just by being available to be identified with in the very grain of one's illness (which is to say, the grain of one's own intellectual, emotional, bodily self as refracted through illness and as resistant to it)—being available for identification to friends, but as well to people who don't love one; even to people who may not like one at all nor even wish one well. All of these may nonetheless be brought consciously, even if haltingly, into the world of people living with this disease—just as, whatever one's privilege, a person living with fatal disease in this particular culture is inducted ever more consciously, ever more needily, yet with ever more profound and transformative revulsion into the manglingly differential world of health care under American capitalism. It's been one of the great ideological triumphs of AIDS activism that, for a whole series of overlapping communities, any person living with AIDS is now visible, not only as someone dealing with a particular, difficult cluster of pathogens, but equally as someone who is by that very fact defined as a victim of state violence. What needs to happen now, and I believe can happen, is the even more radical and shaming realization that under the present regime of systematic exclusion from health care in at least the U.S., *every* experience of illness is, among other things, a subjection to state violence, and where possible to be resisted as that.

10.

One of the first things I felt when facing the diagnosis of breast cancer was, "Shit, now I guess I really must be a woman." A lot of what I was responding to was the way the formal and folk ideologies around breast cancer not only construct it as a secret, but construct it as the secret whose sharing defines women as such. All this as if the most obvious thing in the world were the defining centrality of her breasts to any woman's sense of her gender identity and integrity! This did not happen to be my situation: as a person who has been non-procreative by choice, and whose sense of femininity, whatever it may consist in, has never been routed through a pretty appearance in the imagined view of heterosexual men—as a woman moreover whose breast eroticism wasn't strong—I was someone to whom these mammary globes, though pleasing in myself and in others who sported them, were nonetheless relatively peripheral to the complex places where sexuality and gender identity really happen. Something similar has seemed true, moreover, to many other very different women I have talked with, including the other women who sat angrily through a meeting of the hospital-organized breast cancer support group, being told by a social worker that with proper toning exercise, makeup, wigs, and a well-fitting prosthesis, we could feel just as feminine as we ever had and no one (i.e., no man) need ever know that anything had happened. As if our unceasing function is to present, heterosexually, the spectacle of the place where men may disavow their own mortality and need as well as ours. But how different was this, after all, from the message I heard a week before the diagnosis, at an "evening of wit, wisdom, and storytelling for lesbians" by Joanne Loulann, whose hilarious, community-healing, butch/femme-celebrating, powerfully sex-affirmative performance was gored by the ugliness of a single moment when she invidiously compared the paucity of federal research money available to "us" (for research into "our" disease, breast cancer) to the supposed riches being poured into research for AIDS. As though AIDS research were choking on excess of resources!—as though AIDS were *not* a disease of women, of lesbians!—but also as though the identity and solidarity of this lesbian-defined audience depended breathlessly on the intimacy of our association with that-disease-that-is-not-AIDS. As though what we all are, as women, butch, femme, androgynous alike, is nonetheless not only the thing defined by breasts but also that-thing-that-is-not-man, that is not the male labeled queer, that thing not vulnerable through poverty or racism, through injection, through an insertive or hot and rubbed-raw sexuality to the bad luck of viral transmission.

The invidious comparison has now become a hurtful commonplace, but many of us in the audience were shocked, hearing it then. I feel I must refuse to identify as a woman on this ground. As a woman, I certainly could contract HIV. I happen to have contracted another, also very often fatal disease that makes its own demands of a new politics, a new identity formation. As a woman, I have been intimately formed by, among other things, the availability for my own identifications of men and of male "perversion," courage, care, loss, struggle, and creativity. I also know that men as well as women have been intimately formed by my and many other women's availability for identification in these ways, and are likely to be even more so in the future. In the day-to-day experience so far of living with and fighting breast cancer, meanwhile, I feel inconceivably far from finding myself at the center of the mysteries of essential femaleness. The people to whose exquisite care I can attribute my present, buoyant spirits and health are the same companions, students, friends, of *every* gender and sexuality, who have always been as vital to my self-formation as I think I have been to theirs. Beyond that, a dizzying array of gender challenges and experiments comes with the initiations of surgery, of chemotherapy, of hormone therapy. Just getting dressed in the morning means deciding how many breasts I will be able to recognize myself if I am wearing (a voice in me keeps whispering, *three*); the apparition of my only slightly fuzzy head, facing me in the mirror after my shower like my own handsome and bald father, demands that I decide if I would feel least alienated or most adventurous or comforted today as Gloria Swanson or Jambi, as a head-covered Chasidic housewife, as an Afro-wannabe in a probably unraveling head rag, as a drag queen who never quite figured out how to do wigs, as a large bald baby or Buddha or wise extraterrestrial, or as—my current choice—the befezzed disciple of my new gay fashion gurus, Akbar and Jeff. Indeed every aspect of a self comes up for grabs under the pressure of modern medicine, with its strange mix of the most delicate and the coarsest of knowledges and imaging capabilities. That pretty, speckled, robin's-egg blue pill with the slightly sinister name "Cytoxan"—it was indeed developed during the Second World War as a chemical warfare agent; when, as per doctor's instructions, I drop four of this "agent" into my bloodstream every morning, the *mildest* way to describe what is happening is via the postmodernist cliché that I am "putting in question the concept of agency"! I have never felt less stability in my gender, age, and racial identities, nor—anxious and full of the shreds of dread, shame, and mourning as this process is—have I ever felt more of a mind to explore and exploit every possibility.

11.

There's so much to be said about the powerfully performative rhetorical force of obituaries and memorials. How can I even think about the task of writing an obituary for someone who's alive? I tell myself sometimes that being sick has made me read obituaries differently, but really I have always been fascinated by them in the same "morbid" way, I have always propelled myself into all the positions around every obituary I saw with the whole force of this particular imagination. My own real dread has never been about dying young but about losing the people who make me want to live. For many other people these things arrange themselves differently; but all are wrung, whirlpooled, turned inside out in the obituary relation. The most compelling thing about obituaries is how openly they rupture the conventional relations of a person and of address. From a tombstone, from the tiny print of the *New York Times,* from the panels on panels on panels of the Names Project quilt, whose voice speaks impossibly to whom? From where is this rhetorical power borrowed, and how and to whom is it to be repaid? We miss you. Remember me. She hated to say goodbye. Participating in these speech acts, we hardly know whether to be interpellated as survivors, bereft; as witnesses or even judges; or as the very dead. I look at my snapshots from the 1987 gay and lesbian march on Washington—I see Michael across a distance, white glasses blazing, looking young and forlorn with no mustache; it's only weeks after Bill's sudden death; in the panels of the quilt, I see that anyone, living or dead, may occupy the position of the speaker, the spoken to, the spoken about. When the fabric squares speak, they say,

"Love you! Kelly."

"Frederic Abrams. 'Such Drama.'"

"Roy Cohn. Bully. Coward. Victim."

"Michel Foucault. Where there is power, there is resistance...a plurality of resistances...spread over time and space....It is doubtless the strategic codification of these resistances that makes a revolution possible."

"For our little brother, David Lee."

"Sweet dreams."

"Hug Me."

Churned out of this mill of identities crossed by desires crossed by identifications is, it seems—it certainly seemed in October of 1987—a fractured and *therefore* militant body of queer rebellion.

But no one can really claim or own the relations of mourning. This winter in North Carolina, an ACT UP friend and I went to do some fence mending with the local Names Project committee—a committee that we sometimes feel is monopolizing, for no purpose more liberatory than memorializing and consolation, the energies and money of a lot of the A-list of North Carolina gays for which we think we could find considerably more telling uses. At what we thought, with relief, was the breakup of a long meeting, the unctuous guy who was chairing the committee announced that, to remind ourselves what the committee was all about and to rededicate ourselves to our (or its) purposes, he and some other people were going to unfold, in the lobby of the building, the latest of the big quilt panels that had passed through their hands—for us to review. I had to do it, but I didn't want to. The quilt wrings me out, as it does any viewer, in a way I don't always want to be available to be wrung out; it was a time when somebody I loved very much was barely hanging on and wasn't sure he wanted to; and just then I was very angry with the project, with its nostalgic ideology and no politics, with its big, ever-growing, and sometimes obstructive niche in the ecology of gay organizing and self-formation. Truculently and furiously I perused, as it unfolded, the random patchwork of other people's mourning, daring it to make me cry (I felt as though I would be lost if I started crying that night)— the now familiar topoi of these terrible losses, the appliquéd rainbows, teddy bears, photographs, baby blocks, 501s; the first-person utterance of survivors, the awful first-person utterance attributed to the dead. I felt, somewhat desperately, as though I knew and could at that moment resist it all. As it turned out, the square I had no way of dealing with was the one appliquéd with SILENCE = DEATH and ACT UP tee shirts: not because of them, but because of the unplaceable, unassuageable voice of its lettering, which said starkly: "HE HATED THE QUILT." I don't know whether my tears and bile were finally those of rage, surrender, envious exultation, or absolute hopelessness. I don't know whose powerful voices I was hearing or which were triumphing: the heroic and now immortalized refusal of the dead man; the—what? I don't know how to begin to characterize the possible tones—of the survivors who honored him and by the same gesture surrendered him up to what he hated; or the ravenously denuding, homogenizing, relentlessly anthropomorphizing and yet relentlessly disorientating abyssal voice of the obituary imperative, the implacably inclusive format of memorial relation and address.

12.

I think Michael is very, very tired of being sick, and I think I can feel that with him—though I also feel that every day that Michael is there and recognizably himself, gossipy, courageous, universally inquisitive, perhaps crabby, communicative, and craving physical touch, is a day that I have an important reason to be happy. My own illness hasn't really even begun to come home to roost—it probably won't for some years, *maybe* never—but I also see, or imagine, some of the people who love me beginning to deal with the possibility that someday the same calculus may operate around my own fatigue, discouragement, pain, flares of zest and creativity, the recognizable, recognizing, and hurting shards of relation and identity. I still want to know more and more about how Michael and other people deal with this long moment, and about how I will. As whom, as what I may deal with it; out of what spaces I may speak of it, or be spoken for in these identities and struggles—I know these are not simply for me or even for my immediate communities to decide; yet I relish knowing that enough of us will be here to demonstrate that the answer can hardly be what anyone will have expected.

13.

A week ago at a country inn on Lake Huron, Michael and another friend and I were talking about White Glasses ("White Glasses" the talk, not white glasses the glasses). Michael said—perhaps apprehensively—"I'm certainly glad I'm not going to be there."

I said—*distinctly* apprehensively—"I'm certainly glad you're not going to be there, too. But I still want you to get a kick out of this."

"Oh, I *am*, I am," Michael said. "Are you going to record it for me?" So I am recording it. Hi Michael! I know I probably got almost everything wrong but I hope you didn't just hate this. See you in a couple of weeks.

Notes

Michael Lynch died of AIDS on July 9, 1991.

[1] Michael Lynch, "Tobacco," *These Waves of Dying Friends* (New York: Contact II Publications, 1989), p. 65.

[2] Butler writes "has been refused"; I have chosen to bracket the word "been" to record the effects of her notation that "Lacan fails to make clear who refuses whom" (Butler, *Gender Trouble,* pp. 49-50).

[3] Michael Moon, "Memorial Rags, Memorial Rages," unpublished draft. I am very grateful for the opportunity to see this draft and permission to quote from it.

[4] The best sample of this in writing is Michael Lynch's "Last Onsets: Teaching with AIDS," in *Profession* 1990: 32-36.

Carole Simmons Oles

Lateral Time

I AM STANDING IN THE LAUNDRY ROOM AT University of Alaska Southeast in Juneau. The washers and dryers spin, sending up a cacophany of zippers clashing with steel, blades thrashing fabric. The phone on the wall is adjacent to these machines and the Coke and Fritos dispensers, which in drawing electric power contribute their own racket of monotonous humming.

Leaning against the wall with one finger in my right ear while the other adheres to the receiver, I am trying to hear a nurse in Northern California tell me the truth about what a doctor there, self-proclaimed breast specialist, described to me as a twenty-minute procedure. The nurse is telling me how someone must accompany me, that I will be given Valium, that I will lie on my stomach on a table with a hole in it through which my left breast will dangle while the radiologist performs a stereotactic needle biopsy on me to determine the nature of "suspicious" microcalcifications, which have been observed, sonogrammed, observed again on film, and possibly have increased in number since first spotted and shown to me, innocent looking specks, white dust on a black x-ray ground. She is telling me more than I want to know.

Her description of the process itself takes almost twenty minutes, and as she speaks I find myself becoming more and more anxious, feel myself spinning around in the medical care machine, which has never before so ominously threatened to clean me. The nurse and I are talking about the one day I can possibly have this procedure, between my teaching in Juneau and my second stint of the summer, in Rowe, New Mexico. We have scheduled a time, and now I can't wait to get off the phone.

The hometown breast expert had told me before I left for Alaska that this was probably nothing, that roughly 30 percent of these biopsies came back malignant and he gave me a 10 percent chance. So I didn't feel any rush. He'd also said that if it did turn out to be cancer, probably it would be another ten years before it developed into anything of consequence. To whom? I wonder in retrospect... He'd said many things I had occasion to question.

A few days later I phone back the nurse to say I will schedule the biopsy at the end of the summer, after my return from New Mexico. Amid the grandeur of the Alaskan landscape, I try not to think about it. I know I am small, and Alaska tells me so resoundingly. Much smaller than the white periods on my x-ray.

June 7, 1997. Tracy Arm Fjord, en route from Juneau: low-flying scoters, water every shade of green, humpback whale beside the stilled boat, bald eagles, south face of Sawyer Glacier: 300 feet high, 300 feet under water; 20 miles back fed by Sukeen snow/icefield of 1250 square miles. North face: since 1988 receded as shown by pale rock where vegetation hasn't yet grown; lichen first, then others. Around the south face, on every floe, a mother sea lion with her pup. We tread lightly, cut the engines so as not to frighten them. They look up from their drowse, a scene more pristine and pure than any I've ever witnessed. The passengers go utterly silent.

June 15. En route to Gustavus: entering Icy Strait, a striking presence, the Fairweather mountains, entirely snow-covered and craggy, being pushed up by two contending geologic plates. So many bald eagles! In one binocular span, three: one atop a rock on a small island, two farther onshore, in two trees. And a humpback glimpsed earlier: a huge presence to our right, between two small boats which stop dead. No wonder!

Later, change of plan: we can't reach Gustavus—the dock is under a four-foot tide and winds over twenty knots, so we head farther on, to Bartlett Cove. Wildlife tour canceled. Sailing back to Juneau, we encounter more whales and a towed barge loaded with containers labeled "Spill Response Equipment."

Flying out of Juneau, we're delayed by fog. I can't make my connection to California, must spend the night in Seattle and return home late afternoon next day—the day I was to have had the biopsy I canceled.

At home, Chico, California, June 23. I call the radiologist; if I pick up the film from his office, he'll discuss it with me—the "Possible increase in the number of calcifications within cluster seen in mid aspect of left breast. Difficult to be sure due to differences in technique." It's the "differences in technique" I want to hear about before submitting to the procedure the nurse has candidly described.

I talk to her again and she explains the language of the mammography report as "a general disclaimer they use" because from one technician to another elements of the exam will differ. She helps me determine what questions to ask: what is the level of suspicion? On that basis, how much leeway do we have in diagnostic procedures (i.e., time)? What is safe for me? Spill Response Equipment...

June 24, New Mexico. A restive night—turned in at 9:30 exhausted and proceeded to hear voices, cicada chorus, and rumblings inside my own head, for what seemed another couple of hours. Then, early this morning, disturbing dreams of not being able to find my way to classes, in a strange city wanting to ask directions of students and always taking the wrong turns, winding up at one point in an abandoned, scary cave of a place. In one frame, my friend since third grade, Phyllis, is very ill. When I fitfully half-wake, I have trouble breathing. Altitude.

Aspens and poplars through one long, narrow window, tossing coins at me. Long after I leave they will reveal their true gold. Weather more troubled today, a cast of gray in the sky's blue and white clouds piling up in boiling heaps. Yesterday was perfect clarity. Oh, for a mind and spirit consistent.

Yesterday in Denver airport, waiting for connecting flight I thought again—struck me in Alaska too—how lucky I am to be able to see such beauty this summer. Lucky I didn't go blind in my right eye when the retina detached last January. And then how even knowledge of, contemplation of, Alaska and New Mexico would have been impossible a hundred years ago—much less standing in both in less than a week. Lateral time, the collapse of barriers and the creation of new relationships—a new simultaneity. Will the physical ability to stand on a given place limit imaginings?—of it, no doubt—but not of other places, yet physically inaccessible. My eyes are burning and the altitude is pressing in on my sinuses, nasal passages, my sleep.

July 6. Thunder rolling around us and conflagrations of clouds boiling up at intervals over the Mesa. Intricate dreams many nights—unrecoverable scenes of travel along precipitous edges, accidents, walking on ice. Strong wind, storms circling, and the basketballs blowing around the tennis court absent any players; one ball making for the open gate in the chain-link fence.

Luci Tapahonso singing in Navajo: "In beauty, it is restored."

Scott Momaday, booming voice like the voice of God in his poems, in dialogue with the bear. From "Berries"—Bear says "Sometimes I'm so lonely I could die." Yahweh says "I am always lonely and I cannot die."

Nan's gold teeth, her broad smiling face reassure me.

September 14, to California. On yesterday's drive to Berkeley, two striking images; first, on 45 beside the immense towers of the Farmer's Rice Cooperative pale yellow baking in the heat, two men—at first indistinguishable as such—frail farmers against those enormous containers. Then on 505 with its gentle, rolling hills devoid of any sign of human proximity save the occasional fence—hills also bleached now, containers for light that has dried them all summer, a solitary llama climbing over the rise, surveying all those acres with the presence and proprietorship of a feudal lord.

Yellow, bleached yellow. The color of the season. Then in Berkeley, a riot of bougainvillea, and too many people on the streets.

September 20. Days and nights spent worrying about breast cancer. The language of these reports "suspicious abnormalities" and medical personnel "he'll make an opening"—you mean an incision?—"an opening"—she resists using the most descriptive word. Wherein lies truth? Whom to trust?

No wonder silence is adopted as a way of life, a way of keeping peace.

I hope to live till Christmas.

September 27. Last night I dream-drove the Juneau Road—from the hill I saw into the far distance mountains layered and at their feet tiny people moving about. Driving that one road, from beginning to end—a life rising from, falling off into water.

October 2. Today sunny with high patchy clouds after last night's strange weather. The TV blasted first, then an hour later the electricity gone in rain, wind. I lighted candles, the oil lamp. Could read by them Cynthia Ozick's "Lovesickness" in an old *New Yorker*—and other tidbits squinted at. Was glad for Walkman; though the radio brought me only religious kooks and heavy metal. Listened to Price and Domingo on tape sing duets from Verdi and Puccini. The natural disturbances an edgy manifestation of my personal physical one. But just before 11 P.M. the power returned. Now, in ten minutes, I leave for the biopsy. Already these last weeks, everything altered...

It's the birthday of Wallace Stevens, hence a reading on NPR of "Postcard from the Volcano"—*smear of the opulent sun* over the field of a mammogram.

At the Breast Center on the outskirts of town, adjacent to a retirement community, the nurses are kind as I'm prepped for the procedure. They all have breasts or appear to and in this context I wonder what may be lurking in theirs as they minister to woman after woman here where floral paintings and restful decor seem rather to increase fear and tension by declaring that we need be distracted from it. In my hospital johnny, I am asked to sign two releases, the second granting permission for insertion of a titanium clip at the site of the biopsy. No one has ever mentioned this to me and I am unwilling to sign, though the physician too asks me as I lie face down on the table, needle inserted in my left breast, to accept this probe. I don't understand why the scar of the biopsy itself isn't mark of the site and again I decline. It will help pinpoint the location of the bad word if pathology finds one. If... I say, I'll have a mastectomy. This seems to surprise him but I have already tallied the legion of friends who've endured mastectomies and I see myself joining them if cancer blooms in my breast. I am not yet making fine distinctions. The biopsy is no small matter to her with the needle inserted; the target feels more than she wants to. She wishes this were over before it is, the awkward position, the palpable punching and sucking out of tissue. Like a woman in a bad joke, I go home and take two Tylenol.

October 3. Afterthoughts re the titanium clip/probe: No, you're not going to plant a flag on me like the moon. I'm not part of your space exploration. This country has a mind of her own. No surprise parties, no "presents" like your titanium staple manufactured by a large reputable company. Stick it.

October 6. The day a voice on the phone (which I have had to call for results of the biopsy) tells me I have ductal carcinoma in situ.

Everything had already changed and now instead of waiting to hear if I am the one or the seven, I focus on what happens next: what questions to ask, whom to tell, how to keep working; and what of my daughter? sister? I drag them with me into a different column...and immediately leave for my teeth-cleaning appointment, head thick, mind weighed down with the news, with the new territory I enter, being the one out of some eight, knowing my friend one of the lucky seven—when she told me the results of her biopsy a week ago I felt my odds shift. The new dental hygienist is awful, avid listener to the poetic essays of Kay Trumbull. Her hands lean on my face, my eye, her arm presses on my right breast—Get off me! I want to yell. The doctor for one reads the message when I say the news of a cracked tooth, imminent new crown isn't my first or worst news of the day—he for one doesn't press the mirror on me to examine another cracked tooth when she urges me to and I insist, No!

Home under gunmetal skies, in wind and rain: the "pathetic fallacy" but yes it is nature enacting the darkness that falls over my life. Into a flannel nightgown, the shawl from my dear friends in Vermont around me, and into bed, hoping to sleep just a little before I grade papers, hoping to repair the deficit. Nothing doing.

Get up, write e-mail to all who know about the biopsy. My son calls, worried. We talk information, as much as I can give. Then my daughter, who is shocked, says she thought the "question" would be nothing. We laugh—Amazons knew to kick butt—we're sad, we too share information. She's pleased with fine photos her brother has taken of her new baby, blessed news of the healthy. Then my Vermont friends call—a long talk, details, questions and some answers.

How will they see me tomorrow at school? As differently as I now feel and see myself? Mortality sticking out like quills.

October 4, consultation. As I sit in the waiting room of Dr. X's office, pretending to fix my mind on the magazine in my hands, I overhear the receptionist on the phone with a patient—on the other end, Velma is not seeming to get what the receptionist is saying, growing impatience edges her voice until, exasperated, she asks to speak to Velma's husband. Suddenly the receptionist's tone changes as she says, "Oh, *that* Velma." She's been looking at another patient's records while she spoke. Anyone can make a mistake, I'm thinking; at the same time it seems unlikely, cruel even, to mix up two Velmas. Then I am moved into one of the examining rooms where I sit at the far end by the window, at the foot of the table, *Dr. Susan Love's Breast Book* and a notepad of questions on my lap. Some minutes later the door opens, and Dr. X enters, closing it behind him. He pulls up a chair and wheels it as far as possible from me, up against the door.

He lists several alternative courses of treatment, doesn't want to be interrupted. Twice he excuses himself and goes, I imagine, to see another patient, the second time leaving the room ringing with his "You can read your book." My uneasiness is mounting and it has not to do with the urgency of my physical situation but the manner in which I am being treated by this de facto (default?) expert. A short time later he's back again, and quite tired of my list of questions. Now I breathe deeply and—against all the manners and medico-hero-worship of my upbringing—confront him: he must not be impatient with me, must answer my questions, must realize how emotional and frightening this is for me. If he has no time to answer my questions now, I'll come back another day.

Aha. Thus challenged, in a single push he wheels his chair too close to me and begins to draw me pictures on his pad. If his obvious wish to escape the room was unsettling, this hostile proximity is even more so. Soon I'm out of there and standing beside him at the receptionist's desk; it will be up to me to call back when I've decided what treatment option to follow. I will never keep my word to come back another day, but I don't know that yet. Nor do I know, until I talk to nurses at the Breast Center as

I'm assembling records for treatment at UCLA, that Dr. X had not seen the pathology report of my biopsy when we had our last consultation. This may explain much of his behavior, though surely not excuse it. Nor would it explain his definitive statement, "Write this down: size is not important in DCIS." Important for what? It helps determine course of treatment, I had to learn elsewhere.

Postscript re Dr. X: a few days after the office visit, I receive a note on pink stationery, reading: "Dear Carole, Please pardon my impatience that I displayed on your last visit. I do appreciate the stress you are undergoing and the frustration of trying to understand the compexity [sic] of your disease. Much of it has to be digested over time as it is, otherwise, overwelming [sic]. In the end, it will become simplier [sic]. Sincerely, Dr. [X]."

During the period between diagnosis and treatment, I do not write about what's happening to me for the most part, barely have time to talk to several people about it. I am suddenly amazed at the number of women, women I do and don't know at the university alone, willing to discuss their own experiences with breast cancer. My energy must be conserved for taking care of myself and doing my job. Anything else has to be jettisoned. I make myself scarce, try to stay calm and unstressed. I take my vitamins more faithfully than before. Everything around me blurs. I plunge into problem-solving mode: out of my way, everyone. Maybe I can do it and maybe I can't but you can't distract me. Immersion is my style. The minute I decide never to walk into Dr. X's office again, I feel better.

October 12. All week breast breast breast breast breast and allied subjects doctors treatments x-rays glass slides substandard care advocacy and more ad infinitum.

My favorite breast! The laundry hanging in the bathroom yesterday—all those bras with two chambers. After a typically wakeful night, lying in bed this morning till nearly nine as if staying there, nodding off, I'll wake and it won't be true—if only I stay in bed long enough.

And the snippet of dream, in which my daughter flanked by my mother and me says, "I see my complete Mommy is here."

I talk to two actor friends in Rhode Island. The woman has heard of Dr. Susan Love, having read her book when she played in *The Waiting Room* by Lisa Loomer, in which one character has breast cancer. I tell the man I'm reading someone I can trust, Dr. Susan Love, for enlightenment, guidance, and honest, humane talk. He's never heard of her, but several nights later he calls having read of her in *The Advocate*, local gay paper, and tells me she's appearing on Lifetime TV. We're both intrigued to learn that she set out to be a nun before going to medical school.

The wise voice that helps me through this time is Dr. Love's. When I read of the Multidisciplinary Clinic at UCLA, her new bailiwick, modeled after the one she established at Boston's Faulkner Hospital, I know I've struck gold. I ferret out the phone number from Information and, to my amazement, can make an appointment for the next week. Later the logistics of getting there, providing for my classes, keeping things up in the old life even as I enter the new one. At each stage of this process, though, I feel more secure as I decide to seek what seems some of the best care available anywhere.

A friend offers to fly with me to Los Angeles, but I decline on the principle that I may need her more later. It's easy enough to drive to Sacramento, fly nonstop to L.A., where my sister's friend will meet me at the airport, introduce me to her leonberger dog, Cosmo, drive me around Westwood, have brunch with me, and generally distract me from my purpose. After the noon to 5:00 clinic, I will have to spend the night at Tiverton House, the nonprofit residence operated by UCLA primarily for use by patients at the university's numerous medical facilities. I will see from some other guests that I am now truly in the world of the ill, despite the palm trees, golden light, soft air.

*

October 17. I sit with six other women in the waiting room at UCLA's Multi Clinic. At 12:20 P.M., one of us says, "The fun begins..." as she fills out the forms the rest of us have already submitted. We are all ages: one woman is accompanied by her husband, who moves with a walker, one is a young mother in her twenties. Carmen has taken our vital signs, then sent us back to this discreet corner of a larger waiting room. I have already given permission for any number of takeovers: surgery or other procedures deemed immediately necessary; records disclosed as deemed necessary; financial matters disclosed to lawyers in the event of etcetera. Another husband joins us: tall, Asian, very handsome with gray hair well-styled and a bottle of spring water dangling from his left hand. He looks worried. How do I look? The woman filling out forms is wishing out loud that it were five o'clock and she could go home; the younger woman beside her—a daughter?—strokes her arm.

As I await the arrival of Dr. Y, my surgeon who will report on the Multidisciplinary committee's recommendations for me, I am reading Emerson's "Self-Reliance": *O father, O mother, O wife, O brother, O friend, I have lived with you after appearances hitherto. Henceforward I am the truth's.*

Each of us is assigned her own room, with some reading material and the tape recorder on a table against the wall, ready to preserve for later replaying the panel of experts' recommendations for treatment. The panel consists of surgeon, oncologist, psychologist, radiologist. The room is cold and I get a blanket to wrap around me. Still, the air-conditioning in here is excessive, and by the end of four hours I have a sore throat. The door is left ajar, and first I am assigned one surgeon, then another. It seems I will only be visited by a nurse, the psychologist, and the surgeon. Other women in adjacent rooms have a different panoply of visitors, suited to the particulars of their breast cancers. I hear the woman next door say she is still surprised when she must utter these two words to describe herself. Like the rest of us, she can't quite believe this is happening.

When Dr. Y at last appears, he tells me in a matter of minutes what the group recommends for me: surgical excision. He announces, "Our pathologist would agree with the diagnosis there which says it's cribriform type." When I note that the original report says "*predominantly* cribriform," he counters, "Well, that's semantics" but adds at once, "I'm sorry—you're an English teacher" and goes on to convey more information. While ductal carcinoma in situ is noninvasive (the good news), it is also less simple to excise, given the breast's network of ducts winding and intersecting, potentially hiding more cancer in another segment of duct outside the area of biopsy and surgery. They haven't sent the radiologist to see me on this visit because they are not recommending radiation unless comedo cells are determined present and/or the tumor is greater than one centimeter (half an inch) in size. I tell Dr. Y that I had decided to have a mastectomy rather than radiation, and he states clearly that although they will treat me as I request, they would consider that excessive for what they can observe of my cancer. He is brisk and friendly, willing to answer questions but capable of forestalling them. He tells me to call anytime, and take a week to decide what I want to do. Then it's over and I'm out into the sunshine of Westwood, buses carrying people home from their jobs, students crossing at Westwood and Leconte, strange light I feel around my own body.

Back home, I take three days to decide to follow the Multidisciplinary group's plan. If I need a mastectomy, that can come later. What will be most telling now, as Dr. Y and the nurse both reiterated, is the the pathology report following surgery. I phone Dr. Y and set a date for my return to UCLA. I try to schedule it after a planned reading trip to Pennsylvania in late November, but when he asks, "You want to wait that long?" I change my mind.

These three weeks pass in a fog. I'm touched when several friends offer to accompany me to L.A. for surgery—two from New England—and I'm grateful but need to save them for worse, or at least what I imagine might await me, worse than I've been prepared for. A membrane separates me from the world and my kind. Am I not born yet? I do not want to discuss it, except with a few close friends. I feel ashamed as well as scared, the focus of wrong attention, losing control over my body, my life. The previous January a detached retina, now more decomposition. I am not good at asking for help, do not like to be dependent so I continue to gather information, deliver lectures about statistics—the others. Come, November 3. Let time evaporate, the thing be done.

November 3. Pacing away five more minutes before setting out from Tiverton House. Hot already in L.A., but I will carry a jacket anticipating frigid examining rooms and hours in them.

Dread arrives in many forms: the surgery itself—knife slicing through layers; the findings—what may lie behind the apparent resident in one duct; the aftermath—pain, potential problems of bleeding and/or infection. And the longer wait afterwards, the huge continuing unknown.

"Traveler Safety Tips" stares at me in red from a list of instructions about crime in hotels. I am a traveler and safety slips away through locked doors.

November 7. Wrapped in a blanket, in my comforting bed at home. Wanting to stay away from school from all human contact. Want to stay horizontal. Yesterday, lying on the couch resting before setting out to try to teach Women Writers course, imagining myself sharing my story with students and surprised to start crying at my own news as if hearing it for the first time myself. Now, in decisions and actions taken—at least temporarily—I recognize with my whole awareness that I have/had cancer. In my file drawer I keep bills in a folder labeled "BC." I don't want *cancer* sitting in there among the everyday, don't want it to exist any more than I wanted to see the large flat envelope full of mammograms or the FedEx envelope stuffed with my bubble-wrapped glass slides.

8:21 A.M. I write on the sign-in sheet at the surgical center on Monday, November 3, 1997. I am early even after sitting in the lobby and reading the L.A. paper, after visiting yet another restroom. In the waiting area, other women accumulate, some with women friends, some with spouses. I read or appear to read *Nature Conservancy*, traveling up and down the Virginia/Maryland spit of land out into Chesapeake Bay—Nassawadox my favorite name, the one I revisit, waiting. Finally I'm called.

I follow Marie into the serious rooms behind the desk where I signed in. Rows of curtained cubicles where we are prepared for whatever form of breast surgery brings us here today. Some of us will leave without breasts—others, we hope, merely without cancer. But even we know enough now to see the folly of this hope, the conditional status we now occupy in our own bodies on earth. Marie asks me medical history questions. Everything of real consequence seems to have happened to me long ago: tonsillectomy, stopping smoking, having a seizure after a head injury, having children, stopping periods. So long ago I mix up even decades, not just years within them. I am instructed to take off everything, even my paternal grandmother's diamond stud in my right ear. My belongings now belong in a plastic bag issued by the hospital, soon to be secured in a locker assigned me. What I must wear instead is sterile, disposable, or allowing easy access to my body, all of it, which steadily becomes now the provenance of others as I retreat deeper inside it to someplace I can remain unobserved and safe. This arm? this haunch?—sure, all yours. No matter if the flap opens—it's not *me* who shines out in her marbled flesh, just a demonstration of flesh itself, generic and unremarkable. I am allowed to keep my glasses—a

name label stuck to the ear piece, since this item among all others most frequently gets sucked into the system, never again to
surface. Now Marie tires of me and pulls the curtain aside to
ready a wheelchair—wheelchair!—for my journey to the basement for the localization procedure that precedes surgery. A man
whose name I miss takes over here. I ask why I need a wheelchair—this bothers me—but there's no talking anyone out of
anything now.

So. Out of this friendly area where all of us wear the same
paper shoes and revealing shifts. Into the corridors, past people in
heavy fabric, people who glance up from their magazines to watch
the sick one pass. I try to look straight ahead. I try not to be the
one in this chair. Out then to the elevators, and a 180-degree turn
for Sonny to back me onto the elevator. At first we're alone in it
and I try to assert who I really am by telling him he's a good driver. But my effort falters when the elevator stops between 6 and
basement to let in people tall on their own feet. Again I stare hard
at nothing, the aspect of the blind. We arrive finally and I'm
brought out frontways, curved sharply to a door Sonny opens,
pushed into a waiting room, very small, where people sit on
chairs close to me—no possibility we can't see each other. We're
through it fast and into a place where uniformed nurses, radiolo-
gists pass with certitude.

Now I'm in Stella's seemingly capable hands. She's a large, dark
woman with a full red smile and operates the LoRad mammogram
machinery—a torturer of sorts but only out to map me for the surgeon. She's his runner, his advance guard. Without her, he's lost in
me. She photographs profusely my interesting left breast. In fact
this, my favorite breast, has never received such careful attention
from any adult. She gets some good shots but needs greater magnification so takes more, each time making me hold my breath
even as she admits she can't exactly say why this is required. Finally
she gets the photos she wants and now two other women arrive to
proceed with the next part.

One has spoken to me in advance of the whole procedure about just what they'll be doing—I needed to sign for her, too (I've given my name away so many times today I wonder will any of it be left for me)—and the other is a radiologist, a full-fledged physician who seems to be training or at least guiding the other. They are going fishing inside my breast. Their lines are wires, with little barbs on the ends, which will be attached when they find just the places they want to catch for the surgeon to pull out. This is far more attention than a breast is destined to have. I hear the word hematoma, once from the next room and once from the radiologist now positioned behind me and I think guiding the technician who stands at my left, doing her infernal casting. A cylinder of plastic in front of me on the machine is placed perfectly to keep my head from moving at all; even if I wanted to disobey the doctor's order to "Don't look" I couldn't. The hematoma seems to be what's causing us all such consternation but we don't give up and finally the wires are sunk.

Stella sticks some markers on me, paints me with dye like a slide, then bandages me and ever so lightly inks x's on spots where, under the bandage, the wires await the surgeon's admiration. Several times during the more unfriendly parts of this procedure, one or the other—Stella or the doctor—pats my shoulder or asks how I'm doing. But I am only being done. I'm glad when Stella passes me on to my new driver but sorry to leave her large comforting presence and her smile. Oh mama.

Now I am really doing this. Okay. Let's get it finished. The anesthesiologist visits me when I'm back in my cubicle on the sixth floor. A medical student, female, comes first to take more medical history. I think she's repeating Marie, but I see that her questions require more evaluative, less factual answers: she writes sentences and paragraphs rather than check-marks or dates. Though she wears the same ubiquitous sterile duds, she has a cough and sniffles. Get her away from me! Now Dr. Anesthesia. Chatty. Where do I teach? Telling me his daughter is studying writing at San Diego State. Telling me I'll be getting twilight sleep, a state between local and general anesthesia. Not what I'd been told to expect, but at this point I am only submitting. He doesn't like the vein in my left hand that though prominent enough seems, quite sensibly to me, to be resisting his attempts to pierce it. At last, success, and he begins circulating through me what I will only later find more like 3:00 A.M. than twilight sleep. Dr. Y is last in with forms to sign. A moment of searching to recall the town I have come from, but bingo. And funny, one of the "risks" of surgery he's listed to discuss with me is "scar." Is there ever not a scar? Or is everything beginning to seem bizarre now, with Dr. Sleep's stuff sliding over my mind? He asks someone, Can we get into surgery early? A phone call, the word, and off we go; I don't know who's pushing me now. We sweep into the O.R., previous crew just barely folding up their tents, complaining a little to the brash newcomers. I levitate from gurney to table with a crowd around for the spectacle, I guess Dr. Y is out there somewhere. I'm Semele now, cut up and claimed: someone gets my left arm onto a blue foam pillow, someone else gets my right onto another. Someone pushes more blue foam under my legs and the last thing I know the ultimate someone gives me a plastic mask and I'm the disappeared, to myself.

Awake in the recovery room, the more I get to be myself the more nobody I am. Where's that gang that found me the center of its universe? Abandoned now!—to one nurse intermittently in the recovery room. Monitored instead by a white plastic clothespin and a self-taking blood pressure cuff that swells every fifteen minutes. I progress toward being boring again. The surgeon appears, maybe for three seconds, and I think I ask him how things went, also think he doesn't answer me, scurries away not to be seen again until—I learn in a half-hour when I am wheeled to a phone to call Rhonda downstairs in the Revlon/UCLA Breast Center to find out when my post-op exam is scheduled—

Tuesday, November 11. Rather a long time to find out what's under the bandage written instructions tell me should remain on for a week.

Four days after surgery, late today more numerous stirrings within—healing, I want to think—some sensation around or near or on the nipple and since I can't see I wonder if it still exists. Only natural to think Dr. Y may have found more than hoped; anything seems possible now that the first thing has befallen: invasive mass not seen on mammogram etcetera.... His non-communication seems only to increase the likelihood. Between emergence from the recovery room and this evening, Friday, when I pick up my pen to finish what started earlier—the long head-splitting night, the many phone calls, the visit with friends, the endless trip back on United Airlines, the aborted attempt to spend a full day at school—between, that is, the euphoria of having surgery over and the recognition that all else only now begins, here I stay trying to keep warm.

> *Wir wandeln durch des Tones Macht*
> *Froh durch des Todes dustre Nacht!*
> *(By the power of music we walk*
> *Cheerfully through the dark night of death!)*
>
> (from the libretto of *The Magic Flute*, act 2, sc. 5, Mozart)

November 9, dream. Last night: in a hospital waiting my turn I go to a bathroom and en route wander into operating rooms packed with bodies. From the corner of my eye, passing one such room: blood pooled on tiles. Bodies on all levels of gurneys, sheets bloodstained. Out into a courtyard where I hope to find my way back to wholeness, but it's the receiving area for bodies being brought in. I turn back into the hospital, past the rooms where someone tells me, "Don't look," but even as the words advise me I see a surgeon holding up an organ, and next a butcher less ceremoniously grabbing a rib roast. I want to get out of this scene, these bodies, but it's the wrong direction, one-way out. I am trying to get back to my waiting mother.

The Princess and the Pea

All night she turns
facing east, facing west
turns herself like a roast
to roll off that pebble
that keeps her alert
uselessly, that knot
over her heart.
Bring on new mattresses
down comforters
mark the spot and don't
at all costs lie on
that speck.
Monsoon rains fill the arroyo
but that pebble stays put
not washing away, not
rolling from under her sleep.
Some princess. No sway
over nuisance the size of a pea.
The last soothsayer arrives
to pronounce in ancient tongue
the cause of no beautyrest
ductal carcinoma in situ.

With a splendid flower arrangement, my daughter sends me one word on a card: "Strength."

November 11. The post-op visit to UCLA starts strangely when I arrive at the surgeon's suite and the receptionist is surprised to see me. Since I have had to fly here from the northern reaches of the state, they make a place for me. I sit in the waiting room first, then in an examining room where a medical student, female, asks me some questions and wants to look at my incision. Of course it is right under the bandage where I was in writing instructed to keep it as dry as possible until this day. Dr. Y is called here and there; messengers keep dropping in to inform me of his progress toward this room. When he at last arrives he cheerfully announces good news from pathology: no comedo cells, a one-centimeter cancer. I like this strategy; it relaxes me for everything else. My medical hero falls slightly off his horse when he is surprised to see I have not removed the bandage. I tell him his written instructions say to leave it on for a week, and he demurs but I don't try to ferret out the paper, which I have in my backpack. He removes the bandage, seems pleased, snips the stitches and places sticky strips on the incision to hold it secure, encouraging the knitting of flesh. I haven't looked at it. Many hours later, in front of my own bathroom mirror I admire the crescent incision above the left nipple, where he disclosed the duct that held the cancer "mid-aspect, behind the nipple," as the radiologist's report described months ago. Now he is urging me to enjoy my trip to Pennsylvania, wishing me luck, wanting a post-op mammogram in two months; and if no further sites are observed, in four months, then six, and six and so on. We part in the corridor outside the examining room and I go outside to the waiting room to look for the sheet of instructions, assure myself that I have not entirely lost my reading comprehension. Just as I find it, Dr. Y passes and I beckon him over, show him the written instructions with his name at the top of the page, the ones that say what he has said they do not. After initial resistance, there is no way of refuting the words on the page before us. I'll have to change that, he says. No sense of victory or satisfaction for me—only the wish that this had not happened, the desire for patients to be able to follow fully the good doctor's clear instructions.

On the phone my friend expresses relief—now that's over and we can get back to normal. Not so fast. You mean you feel more vulnerable? she asks. I *am* more vulnerable, I say. This sums it up. Only the women who have breast cancer don't have this attitude of everything's okay now. It will never be quite okay again. Not to dwell on constantly, but each mammogram and the long-delayed report of results brings fear, each pain forecasts some dire efflorescence. Just after treatment, I begin having a pain in my back, left lung. X-ray reveals nothing. Inside the breast itself, intermittent twinges and pressures, the reassemblage of cells and nerve endings? Months later in the shower I have a sharp, burrowing pain in my left armpit, and alarm bells go off. Each bodily awareness takes its character from cancer—the one that was caught and the one that's running, dodging discovery.

November 26. Hard rains in Chico mean winter begins. Salvia and bougainvillea still blooming, but by morning the blossoms may be strewn on the ground, washed away.

So much fall work deferred—outdoors too. No pruning yet, so this afternoon I see for the first time that Oregon juncos feed on dried lavender seeds—the great bush shakes with four perched there at once, and a fifth on the driveway straining on tiptoe (tip-claw?) to reach the stalks. These juncos wear dark gray, almost black hoods, white shirtfronts, and a blush of sidestripe beneath the wings. How cunning, that one reaching up to be filled. Five years I've lived here, and see them only now. What else do I miss each hour? Rain a cold sound in this poorly insulated house. I struggle against self-pity. This year my body has unfriended me. Yet I must be thankful since it could have been so much worse. And a little voice says, *Just wait . . .* Meanwhile, strength.

December 6, dream. I work at a computer terminal in some school, perhaps Bread Loaf in Vermont, where I teach in the summer, though unaware of others around me. As I type, the screen keeps going dark and then someone tall stands over my left shoulder. I look up to see Bill Matthews, white-haired. He places his hand on mine, a gesture of greeting and friendship. I struggle for a moment—what to say? *I thought you were dead?* I say how happy

I am he's here, I'd heard he was ill. He nods, a slightly crooked smile. Then I'm back at the darkened screen. In that instant of hand-touching, was he here or I there?

Less than a year since diagnosis and treatment, two mammograms following surgery clear, I am teaching in Vermont. When colleagues and acquaintances ask casually about my year, I answer that it's been a hard one. Only if they persist for particulars do I force myself to say, *breast cancer.* A part of me still resists this truth. I also suspect that questioners do not want to hear so much. My mother, who never had breast cancer, died eight weeks ago not of the heart problems we always assumed would overtake her but of a stroke. Maybe death will come at me sidewise too, not where I look for it. Meanwhile, let life come head-on.

Carole Simmons Oles

❧

Interview with
Dr. Susan Love

March 10, 1998

WHEN THE TAXI BRINGS ME TO 845 VIA DE LA PAZ, Pacific Palisades, I think there's been a mistake. The two-story, unimposing white stucco building isn't at all indicative of the doctor's status. But her priorities shine through: on the first floor right, Health Foods Nutrition and Health Products; on the left the Lange Foundation "Miracle Shop"—Pet Rescue Foundation, tax-deductible donations welcomed. Up the flight of stairs, I enter Dr. Love's suite to find her secretary fielding calls and her cocker spaniel settled on the couch in the small waiting room. Through an open door to the inner office I hear Love on the phone where she stays, in animated conversation, about twenty minutes. When it's my turn, I discover her office is almost bare—only the requisite file cabinets, shelves, desk, and a table at which we sit. At first, the dog comes in with us. Love lets her back out into the reception area, presumably to nod off on the couch again. Across the table from Dr. Love, I'm struck by her energy—she's wired, I see her charge zapping off the ends of short black curls. She wears jeans and a sweatshirt, drinks tea and spring water. She amiably reaches over to switch on one of my two tape recorders.

CAROLE SIMMONS OLES: *What made you an advocate for breast cancer when you were a practicing physician?*
SUSAN LOVE: Everybody hopes I will reveal some great revolutionary moment or that I will say my mother died of breast cancer, which she didn't. But actually, what happened was I had

trained as a general surgeon in the times starting out before women's lib when there were very few women in general surgery and the people who did breast cancer surgery were the ones who really couldn't do anything else. Either they were retiring or trying to slow down, or they couldn't do the big operations so they were relegated to breast surgery, which was on the very lowest rung of that hierarchy of what kind of a surgeon you wanted to be. I was bound and determined not to be a breast surgeon because I could do the big operations just like everybody else. Then I went into practice and the only patients I was referred were women with breast problems. It became clear to me pretty quickly that they were being very badly treated and not being given any information. These were still the days of, "Don't worry dear, we'll take care of it." Then you'd wake up without a breast, and nobody had ever discussed anything with you. The breast conservation data was coming out of Italy. We did have American data yet, but we had some pretty good randomized controlled data from Italy. There was an option, but women were not being given it at all. The American surgeons were saying, "Yes, but that data is on Italian women, Italian breasts; we ca believe that." There was an enormous need for someone to talk to women and explain it to them, so that's how I got into it. Around that time I was also looking into the whole notion of fibrocystic disease and in researching that found out how flimsy all of the data was. Every textbook said that if you had fibrocystic disease you had a higher risk of getting cancer. When you tracked it back, it all went to one review paper in the 1950s which was not very good: it really did use scientific principles to compare the data and didn't really define what fibrocystic disease was. My studies showed that fibrocystic disease did not increase the risk of cancer. As I did that research, I realized that women were being badly harmed, both by the lack of scientific rigor and the lack of anybody who would really care for them. That's what really got me involved in breast diseases. And the first wave was taking care of women; I had my own practice, then started the Faulkner Breast Center and a multidisciplinary approach. By that time I really knew how to explain things very well. I did it all day, every day. But that didn't seem to be enough. I felt there were a lot of women out there who were not getting this information from their doctors at all and that's why I wanted to write a book. I had the idea for a while, but I didn't do much about it until I got approached by two publishers around the same time suggesting that I write a book. I realized then that the reason I had not written it is that I hate to write.

I really don't like to write. I talk better than I write.

CSO: *That's where the co-author comes in?*
SL: Right. My co-author, Karen Lindsey, is a poet. She teaches writing at Emerson College in Boston, and she knows nothing about science or medicine at all. I thought about getting a medical writer and then I said no, I could do that part. I don't hate to write quite as much as I did when I started because she's really trained me over the years and I'm better at it than I ever was. The first thing she had to do was teach me not to use the passive voice. In medicine everything is in the passive voice.

CSO: *It's a way of declining responsibility?*
SL: Yeah, the operation was done. The incision was made. There was no one in the room. I have this vision of the knife just sort of floating across the patient.

CSO: *As a reader of the* Breast Book, *one thing I find so engaging is that sense you create in the introduction—"I am going to be holding your hand through this"—without any condescension, and that's what's different.*
SL: The books out there are by people who have been through it, and so it's their story and they throw in a little medical stuff, which is actually plus-minus accuracy because it's filtered through what-

ever they got from the one doctor they went to. Or they're doctors' books, which, no matter how hard they try, tend to be paternalistic or pretty much, "This is what you should do, dear."

CSO: *I think women have been waiting for your book—to grant them the intelligence and power to think about things and make their own decisions and to deal with information. Part of the condescending attitude is, "You can't handle this information."*

SL: You know the most radical thing in the first edition was that I said you had to read your pathology reports. Doctors asked, "What? Why did you put that in?" It makes patients feel so much more powerful. None of these concepts are that hard. It's language. It's vocabulary. If somebody translates it, it's like, "Oh, that's what you're talking about. Of course, I can get that."

CSO: *One thing that writers struggle with is finding time to write. You're a physician, advocate, mother, partner—how do you work it out?*

SL: You steal time from one thing for the other. I don't necessarily sit down and regularly write. I have two books on the back burner that I'll start when I finish business school. So they'll fit into the space I'm now using for homework.

CSO: *That was one of my questions: what's next for you?*

SL: One is another edition of the *Breast Book*, which is ready.

CSO: *What are you adding?*

SL: There's a lot of information to add, a whole new estrogen receptor that we didn't even know existed. There's new hormone stuff, Aridimex, tamoxifen. There are new ways of thinking about how breast cancer works. There's a little bit more gene information now. That's a moving target, but there's more information on that. And we know more about the bone marrow transplant; you can undergo it with fewer problems than I have in the book now, because they've actually gotten better at doing it. The proof that it works hasn't changed, however.

CSO: *Will there be additional information about mapping the ductal structure of the breast?*

SL: I'm getting close to that; I have more information on the anatomy. But I should have that further along by the time I'm writing the next edition. There's more psychosocial information to add. You know, I always think that I'll just change a few chapters and I end up doing everything.

The other book I want to do is how to get your act together in your fifties. This is the follow-up to the *Hormone Book*. The message that became really clear to me doing the *Hormone Book* was that you can do prevention with lifestyle just as well as you can with drugs. Changing your diet, exercising, eating soy, reducing alcohol, and quitting smoking are just as good, and we physicians don't give those as an alternative. And when we do give them we don't tell people how. We say of course you're going to exercise, but we don't say how and where and when, and when you're fifty it is very different from when you're twenty. Not bad or better or worse, but different. I found out last year: I was running and ended up with a shin splint and couldn't do anything for three months. I researched shin splints and found that they're most common in middle-aged, overweight women who push themselves too hard. I said, "Gee, I don't know anybody like that." So I started up again gradually and I was much more into making sure I stretched and warmed up; all kinds of things that are different when you're fifty. What I want to try and do is look into some of the behavior modification literature and really figure out how to help people incorporate these habits into their lives. If you can change your lifestyle, that's the foundation. Then you can choose whether to add drugs or hormones or whatever on top of that. But if you don't have that foundation and you just say, "I'll pop a pill," and then you get breast cancer and can't pop the pill, you're screwed. So we really go at it ass-backwards, in part because the pharmaceutical companies are such a huge lobby and make so much money on it. Anyway, it's not fair to say to people, "I think you should do this" and then not tell them how. I want to try to do that.

CSO: *I'm sure it won't be news for you to hear me say that many women's experience of your writing demonstrates that their doctors fear the* Breast Book.

SL: Because it means the women may know more than they do. And they're scared they don't know enough, which is sort of silly because it's fine. If you come in and say, "Well, I read this," I'll say, "Oh, well, that's interesting, I've learned something new." Now why should that be threatening to me? But they feel somehow that will lower their authority. When I first wrote the book I got a lot of flak in Boston because real doctors don't write popular books. You're translating the mysterious science into English, and it's not something you get points for from your colleagues. I'll bet you a lot of money that most gynecologists don't know the data in the *Hormone Book* either. Not because they're bad or evil but because they're busy, they're seeing a lot of patients, they don't have a lot of time. The meetings they go to are funded by drug companies, and they don't go back and research the original literature.

CSO: *Don't they have scientific skepticism about these things? It seems a great omission.*

SL: No. I've been saying business school is much harder than medical school because in medical school you're not supposed to think. You memorize and hand back. You don't critically evaluate. It's a very different approach, and critically evaluating isn't part of it. So you learn the way to do it and you do it the way you learned.

CSO: *I'd like your reaction to the women's health newsletters as another good source of information.* Our Bodies, Ourselves *was there when we were just beginning to be conscious of these things. Now, these decades later I subscribe to the* Harvard Women's Health Newsletter, *but I feel a little suspicious. Who's making a lot of money from the newsletters?*

S L : Of course! And what is it really about? The real bind is money for projects. It's related to a conversation I had this morning. A group wants to form this American College of Women's Health Physicians but doesn't have a lot of money. There is a lot of money in the pharmaceutical industry; they're dying to give it away.

C S O : *There are strings?*

S L : Sometimes they're not overt strings, which is almost worse. I think it's better if it's a quid pro quo because then you know exactly what you're doing for what. But a lot of times there aren't official strings. If somebody's just given you $500,000 it's harder to criticize them. You know, it's a subtle thing. Now all the medical meetings are funded by the drug companies. All the conferences on women's health are funded by the drug companies, so that the information the doctors are getting is very much filtered through them. The American Heart Association gets a ton of money now from the makers of estrogen. Much of the campaign on women's heart disease is funded by them. Is it bad or good? It's tricky. You do have to be on your guard. I actually think some of these newsletters are worthwhile. I also get the *Harvard Women's Health Newsletter* and I think it's one of the better ones. It's pretty good. The *Women's Health Advocate* is another one I find pretty on-target. And then some of them just rehash without new research.

C S O : *They have the appearance of currency, which can be dangerous.*

S L : Women's health is the newest big market because the health people have finally realized that women make most of the health care decisions in this country. If they can market to women, then women decide where the men get their health care, they decide what operation men and the kids should have. They finally figured out that women are the gateway. All of a sudden we're in the middle and we need to be very careful. For example, Raloxifene is a new hormone approved for osteoporosis; what people are not saying, or what they are saying in the last line of a paragraph of the article, is yes, it's better than a placebo for osteoporosis, but it's not as good as estrogen. It's only half as good as estrogen. Yes, it's somewhat good for lipids, but not as good as estrogen; actually it doesn't increase your HDLs at all, just lowers your LDLs. Yes, it does prevent uterine cancer, which I think is its main selling point. But the breast cancer data is only two years out. It hasn't really been shown to prevent breast cancer, and tamoxifen, which it's modeled after, prevents breast cancer for the first five years and then stops. Raloxifene is going to do the same thing. There's a journal on women's health and they actually had an article written by the president of Wyeth-Ayerst, which makes Premarin, on how wonderful they were because they were opening this research institute on women's health and they were going to study the compliance problem. Why women don't take HRT [hormone replacement therapy] like Premarin. They wrote it like a medical article and it was in the journal as if it were a medical article. It was more like an infomercial. Then the next month there was one written by four people from Lilly, the company that makes Raloxifene, about Raloxifene and how great it was. Again, an infomercial. So we do have to be on our guard. I think there's a pro and a con. It's wonderful that there's so much more information out there, but we always have to be asking where it's coming from and who's gaining from it.

CSO: *Basically we have to have enough studies from impartial sources and ways to disseminate that information. Maybe that would be one of the goals of this new group you mentioned.*
SL: I was talking to them about one thing I'm going to do (I can't do it quite yet): make a think tank on women's health that would really be a conscience for the nation. It's one of my goals, because we do need it. The public is not used to looking at health care information critically the way you do commercials on TV. If you

see a commercial about waxing your floor, you at least think about it, whereas when you see a drug commercial, you don't. Yet they're selling products just the same. Zeneca, which makes tamoxifen, also makes pesticides and bought Sallick, which runs breast cancer clinics. So they're making pesticides, making tamoxifen, and then running the clinics that take care of the cancer patients.

C S O : *They won't lose no matter what happens or who dies of what.*
S L : Of course. From a business standpoint, it's brilliant.

C S O : *This is why you're in business school! Know the enemy.*
S L : It may or may not be the enemy, it's just that we need to be aware of these things. Some people say, "Oh, health care is becoming for-profit." It was always for-profit. You don't think that docs in private practice were there to make money? Of course they were.

C S O : *When I think about the doctors of my childhood, though, things were different; in the forties, say, when I was a kid...*
S L : Because there was less money in this then. Medicare is what did us in. Medicare was when it started to be a way to make money. In fact, it was right at the end of the Second World War when a lot of changes happened. First, with antibiotics it was the first time that you weren't risking your life to be a doctor. That you wouldn't catch polio, TB, bubonic plague, whatever. There was this window of time from the mid-fifties to when AIDS came up. Second thing is Medicare, which was fought tooth and nail by the AMA as socialized medicine, turned out to be the biggest boondoggle that doctors ever had because now they got paid by Medicare for all of the elderly people that got sick. All of a sudden between Medicare and the increase of high-tech science, doctors were making more money. And then there was a third thing, the Vietnam War. You got a deferment if you went to medical school, so a lot of guys went to medical school who would not have become doctors at another time in another place. They were smart

but maybe had different motivations. Might have been in junk bond sales or something like that. Put all of this together, and I think we got what we deserved with managed care. We asked for it as physicians. We were charging high prices. It was wonderful; you could do whatever you wanted to whomever you wanted, charge whatever you wanted and get paid. No quality assurance, no accountability; you never had to prove what you did worked.

CSO: *And now where are we going?*
SL: I think it's going to be better. The potential of managed care is much, much better because you have the demand for accountability, so maybe we can move to evidence-based medicine and away from This-is-the-way-we've-always-done-it medicine, just get rid of the things that don't work and do the things that work. Secondly, get rid of bad doctors. Malpractice suits didn't get rid of bad doctors. You sue people you're mad at, but it doesn't necessarily get rid of the bad doctors. I think quality of care will be better. And with managed care there will be incentive for prevention, which we've never had before. We got paid for treating diseases, for cutting; we got paid for treating you for heart disease, not preventing it. The economics were all to treat diseases. Now the economics have changed and prevention becomes more important. I also think you're going to see many more alternatives. We're already starting to see where the National Cancer Institute says that acupuncture, all of a sudden, has their imprimatur. Why didn't you have alternatives accepted before? Because they were a threat to the doctors. But now the person who's paying, the HMO, wants to get the best care for the cheapest cost. Acupuncture is a hell of a lot cheaper than orthopedic surgery. Whereas in the old system you wanted to do it the most expensive way. You'd much rather operate whether it worked or not. So the change in economics brings a lot of potential. I went to business school because there's a need for people who are bilingual, who can speak business and medicine. The risk is that in trying to fix the abuses of the past,

we go too far in the other direction and forget about taking care of the patients.

CSO: *That's the issue I've been most apprehensive about with the HMOs—denial of care because it costs too much.*
SL: But a lot of what they're denying was worthless. You see, this is the problem: we've spent all of these years convincing the patients that they need too much treatment—because it was to our advantage. Follow-up for breast cancer is a great example. The data is very clear that there is no benefit to blood tests, scans, x-rays after breast cancer. They did a huge randomized control study in Italy, and it showed that the chance of finding metastases earlier and being able to change whether people live or die is zero. But oncologists are doing some of these tests every three months. No data to support that. Absolutely none. What happens then is you get the HMO saying, "We're not going to let you have your blood tests every three or six months" and you feel like you're being deprived. In fact, you were being overtested before. Patients say, "Oh, they're depriving me of getting a bone scan every year" when actually it was worthless and it was only making money for people. HMOs have to find a way to explain that to people. They really can't deny proven stuff. They'd legally be on very shaky grounds.

CSO: *I'm hoping that a lot of the trends that you're talking about really move us in the right direction.*
SL: I think we're going to be much better off, if we make sure managed care fills its potential.

CSO: *I want to shift gears a little to the Lifetime TV interview you did. A gay friend in Providence, Rhode Island, read about it in the* Advocate, *and he knew I was reading your book after my diagnosis, so he phoned and said I had to watch. I've done research on distinguished women of the late nineteenth century, and I'm struck by a pattern of the importance of their fathers in their lives. Would you talk a little about that? I gathered from the TV interview that your father and brother, who were also interviewed, were very supportive of everything you have done.*

S L : I'm the oldest of five—three girls, then a boy, then a girl. I certainly was much closer and more egosyntonic with my father than my mother. I felt I could do whatever I wanted to do, be whatever I wanted to be. I was not pushed, though, at all. My dad didn't go to college; he went to the Second World War, came home, and went to work. My mother didn't finish college. There wasn't this stuff I hear from other people—"Why don't you have all A's and why don't you do this?" My drive was really more internal. But they were certainly supportive of whatever I wanted to do; I always felt that. They were there for me. About the TV show, it was funny. My sisters said, "Oh, we don't want to be on television," and then they were jealous and said, "We should have done it."

C S O : *Another thing, a related question, concerns your Catholicism. I learned from the TV program that you'd been in the convent before attending medical school. In my experience, one of the best traits of Catholicism is its fostering of a sense of moral purpose and of service. I see this very much in you. Does this sound accurate?*

S L : Right, I think you're supposed to give back and leave the world a better place. We're actually now going to the Episcopal Church. I can't bring my daughter up in the Catholic Church. And the Episcopal Church is close enough. They're not homophobic, which helps. The message of giving back is the one I'm very strongly trying to get across to Katie [Love's daughter], too. We did the march on hunger in the Palisades on Sunday and we had a long talk about how it's important not just to give money but also yourself. We wanted to figure out what we could do together. But I agree with you. One of the good things you get from Catholicism is this feeling you really are here for a reason and there's work you need to do to make the world better. We're the grown-ups now, and if we don't make the world better, who else is going to? It was one thing when we were in our twenties and complaining and marching about all the awful things the grown-ups were doing. But now it's our world, we're the grown-ups, so we've got to fix it as best we can.

CSO: *Is there anything you'd like to say that I haven't asked you about?*

SL: I've probably talked my head off. I'm at such a great place right now in my life. I just turned fifty; I love it. You don't have to prove yourself anymore. You sort of did it or you didn't. It's very liberating to be able to plan. That's why I'm saying we're going to see just amazing changes as the baby boomers hit fifty and turn their energies from home and child-rearing to the world at large. If you want to be totally extreme, you can say we need estrogen to domesticate us enough so that we will reproduce the race, and then we get liberated from it at menopause. It makes about as much sense as considering menopause a deficiency. I am looking forward to a huge cohort of postmenopausal women. Unless they drug us all!

CSO: *I hope it's not going to work.*

SL: Oh, I don't think it will work. You know what's very interesting: the new drugs, the Raloxifene and the Fosamax, are what's going to bring down Premarin. Because they've got to make a value proposition, an argument about why you would want to take Ralixofene instead of Premarin. So what is the ad you see in *Parade* magazine for Lilly? Even before Raloxifene came out, they had these ads: if estrogen is so great, why are there still these questions? So now Lilly is fostering all these questions about Premarin. They have these new ads: in *Parade* magazine they show this woman, all these different organs that estrogen is going to help, and then the Raloxifene is called a selective estrogen receptor modulator. Sometimes being selective is not so good. Then you have the Merck Fosamax people who want to take the osteoporosis market away from the estrogen [manufacturers]. So they're fostering questions about estrogen. In a way the marketplace, in fact, is going to be the answer. Premarin has had its monopoly for so long, but now that there's a menu of drugs, all of a sudden people will have to start being honest about what their drug is doing.

CSO: *That's fine, as long as women have the information to make a choice. But if it's just a bigger menu with the same kinds of misleading claims, I'm not sure they'll be much better off. They have to be considering the option of taking no drugs. Your* Hormone Book *will give them a better way of thinking about that.*

SL: That's right. Or if they want to do it, how to do it. Going back to one of your earlier questions, people have said they take my book to the doctor and if the doctor turns pale, they leave. It proves it's the wrong doctor.

CSO: *To close, I wanted to bring you a message from one of the women who's had metastatic cancer, the sister of a friend. When she heard that I was going to have a conversation with you, she said, "Just tell her thank you." So from Pam and all of us, that's the message.*

SL: That's great. But I have to do more! I'm working on research to eradicate breast cancer. We're going to move to something like a Pap smear. We're not going to have surgery or chemo. That's where we're going, that's what I'm working on now. Because I'm tired of taking care of patients one by one. I just want to get rid of the disease. We can't let any more women die!

Amy Ling

Bone Scan

First, they inject a radioactive fluid in your veins
then wait two hours for it to roam your body
—You could set off a geiger counter now, they joke.
Next, you lie on a narrow table and
slowly pass through a large machine
while an image builds gradually on a nearby screen:
first your heel bones, then tarsals and metatarsals, phalanges,
your anklebone, your tibia and fibula...
An hour later your entire skeleton
appears on television
—this is a first—
So that's what you look like!

But then you pause—
how can that be you?
Where are your Asian eyes
yellow-tinged skin,
flat nose,
straight black hair
—all that makes you you,
the cause of so much grief,
eating rice in white bread land,
all that you've finally learned to affirm,
that you're making your living asserting—
all that has disappeared.

Your skeleton looks to you—
untutored in reading skeletal racial signs—
the thigh bone connected to the hip bone—
no better, no worse, no different
from every other skeleton in the world.

Amy Ling

❦

The Alien Within

LABELED A CANCER, HARBORING CANCER, FIGHT-
ing to eliminate cancer—these are all positions—sometimes
sequential, sometimes simultaneous, and always paradoxical—that
I have known.

To begin at the beginning, I am a Chinese American professor
of English born in Japanese-occupied Peiping (as it was called
then) to a mother who was a high school English and music
teacher and a father working on a master's degree in ceramic engi-
neering at Yenching University, a Harvard affiliate. Before my second birthday, we moved to Chungking, the inland wartime capital,
where Japanese bombers followed us. Here, my earliest memories
were of sirens and red balloon air raid signals, damp shelters carved
into the mountainside, bombs exploding buildings and streets into
rubble and craters, bodies mangled and bloodied. In 1944, Father
was selected to be a member of a government scientific team
funded to spend a year in the United States studying ceramic factory methods. The following year, through the help of her adop-
tive mother, a Pennsylvania Dutch missionary nurse to China,
Mother obtained a visitor's visa to the U.S. for herself, my younger
brother, and me.

On November 25, 1945, the army troop transport, for which
we had waited four months in Calcutta, India, slid past the torch-
bearing, giant green lady and deposited us onto a pier in New
York City. Out of the blue, my three-year-old brother asked,
"Whose country is this, theirs or ours?" When my mother

answered, "Theirs," he burst into tears. "Then they'll throw me into the ocean," he cried. In certain ways, his response was uncannily prescient.

When I was nine, our visitors' visas expired and my parents did not participate in the annual Alien Registration required by law each January. The immigration and naturalization officials caught up with us, yanked me out of school (we were living in Mexico, Missouri), and took us to St. Louis to be fingerprinted like criminals. Branded "illegal aliens," we were ordered to return to China. Fortunately for us, before we could be deported, the Communists won control of China and we were reclassified as political refugees and permitted to remain. In 1954, when Asians were finally allowed to become naturalized citizens of the U.S., my family was among the first to claim this privilege.

But having once been labeled "undesirable alien" and "foreign intruder," I have felt my American identity to be a somewhat tenuous thing. Growing up in small towns where we were the only Chinese and during a period when homogenization and assimilation were the goal, I wanted nothing more than to be all-American like my friends. I learned English very quickly (in three months, Mother tells me) and forgot Chinese. I bristled when Father asked why I sang so proudly with the others, "Land of the Pilgrims' pride/Land where my fathers died" when that patently didn't apply to me. I hated being so visibly different and longed for blond hair and blue eyes, the only standard of beauty I knew. Each time I started a new class, curious and outspoken children would ask, "How come your face and nose are so flat?" "Why is your skin yellow?" "How do you Chinese see out of such squinty eyes?" "Do you really sit on the floor and eat with sticks?" I became so self-alienated that I couldn't even say the word "Chinese." It was a term too fraught with embarrassment and humiliation.

It didn't help that Mexico, Missouri was the heart of Little

Dixie. Like the African American poet Countee Cullen, although I also have pleasant memories of that time, one incident stood out and colored everything.[1] Grandma Traub was coming for a visit from Pennsylvania, and Father wanted to treat us all to a dinner at the best restaurant in town. Since Father's income was meager, a dinner out was a rare treat. So I was stunned to see a sign on the restaurant door reading For Whites Only. Father decided to ignore the sign and ushered us all in. I was wishing the floor would open up and swallow us. We seated ourselves and waited for service. Forty-five minutes passed before a waitress brought out menus, then another forty minutes before we received our orders. By this time, the food tasted bitter.

Because the world was so often hostile and I was further handicapped by being socially immature (having skipped two grades), I found refuge in books. When I discovered the public library, I felt like Ali Baba in the robber's cave overflowing with gold and jewels, all there for my taking. I immersed myself in fairy tales, children's classics and found kindred spirits in L. M. Montgomery, Louisa May Alcott, and Jane Austen. As a fifteen-year-old high school senior, I received the highest score in my school on the New York State four-year English Regents exam. So it was natural, when I entered college, that I would want to major in English. However, Father was adamantly against it, insisting, "No one will ever hire a Chinese English teacher." With tremendous effort, I stood up to him and switched my major from Early Childhood Education to English, surprised afterward to find his opposition had melted.

After a B.A. and M.A. in English, I completed a Ph.D. in Comparative Literature at New York University, producing a dissertation entitled "The Painter in the Lives and Works of William Thackeray, Emile Zola, and Henry James." But all the while I felt as though I were diligently jumping hoops someone else had set up; my heart was not engaged. The following poem expresses my feelings about this experience:

```
                  writing
        a dis                sertation
        is like                spinning a web
of your own design                after imbibing several
elephants and conver                ting them to thread.
        Your masterwork            then spans
                  the air
        between two low bushes
        in some narrow byway
        where few people pass.
```

From 1965 to 1969, I taught full time in the SEEK Program at City College of New York with a stellar group of committed young scholars and writers (Toni Cade Bambara, my friend from under-graduate days at Queens College; Mina Shaughnessy; Barbara Christian; Addison Gayle; Audre Lorde; Adrienne Rich). Later, I moved to the SEEK Program at Brooklyn College and in 1972 I went across the Hudson River to be director of Basic Writing at Livingston College, the experimental branch of Rutgers. Working full time, I could study only part time and thus spent ten years completing the doctorate. During this period, from 1965 to 1979, I married, divorced, and married again, and the world also underwent enormous changes.

Looking back on the civil rights and feminist movements, I think of them now as social revolutions as significant as Galileo's discovery that the Earth is not the center of the universe. These movements repositioned the white Anglo-European male—who we had all been taught was the center of the universe—and revealed him to be one of the planets. The rest of us, women and peoples of color, were also planets in our own right, with our own separate orbits all revolving around the same life-giving, nonsectarian sun.

When I realized that I could put my literary training to the task of unearthing women writers who look like me and thereby give a "local habitation and a name" to this interstitial space that previously had no name, I felt I was coming home and coming together in a way that I had never before experienced. My book *Between Worlds: Women Writers of Chinese Ancestry,* the first study ever devoted to this subject, took another decade to bring to fruition, but it was a labor of love. With almost no bibliographic aids and few guides, I dug in this corner of "my mother's garden" by combing shelves of used book stores and the National Union Catalogue under Chinese surnames. Each author I discovered was a jewel to add to my crown.

But when I began this project in the early 1980s, it was an unheard-of and risky thing to do. Because nothing had ever been written on the subject, as far as the Library of Congress Subject Catalogue was concerned, the topic did not exist. Even a friend cautioned me about blazing a trail to a place no one would want to go. During the meeting at which my tenure was discussed, one colleague took notes and reported to me that the professor evaluating my manuscript called it flawed by an "ingrained demureness" and claimed that I'd unearthed only some third-rate authors. His stereotypical and circular reasoning undoubtedly went thus: "She's Chinese; therefore, she's demure. I'm very well read but I've never heard of these authors; therefore, they must be third-rate because if they were first-rate, I would certainly know them." About my poetry, another colleague said, "I don't know much about Chinese poetry, but I don't think much of hers." After the meeting, a colleague who had been a friend explained his lack of support: "We have no Chinese students here, so we don't need a Chinese expert." I asked him how many sixteenth-century Englishmen we had as students; he responded that he didn't wish to pursue that line of reasoning (even though it was his own). I marveled that the poetry critic didn't realize that poems written in English are not "Chinese poems." An African American colleague told me that the discussion focused on defining the central and the peripheral and that the department decided that "criticism can only be done on works that are known, not on works no one has read." Needless to say, I was denied tenure by a humiliating vote. I felt that I was back in front of the restaurant sign: For Whites Only. After a nine-month investigation, I won a grievance suit against my department—not on the basis of bias, however, but on "procedural errors." Winning the grievance gave me only another three-year contract and the "opportunity" to come up for tenure again. I decided to leave instead.

Chinamerican Reflections, my chapbook of poems and paintings, was published by a small press in 1984; *Between Worlds,* my literary history of women writers of Chinese ancestry, appeared in 1990. In those six years, the academic world reversed itself. Though I had lost my personal battle, feminism and multiculturalism were gradually winning the war. In the decade of the eighties, Maxine Hong Kingston's first two books, *The Woman Warrior* and *China Men,* became the most frequently taught books on college campuses by a living American author. In 1988, the Modern Language Association recognized the field by publishing Cheung and Yogi's *Asian American Literature: An Annotated Bibliography,* Amy Tan's *Joy Luck Club* lasted nine months on the best-seller list, and David Henry Hwang's *M. Butterfly* won the Tony Award for best new dramatic play on Broadway. In 1990, I was invited to Harvard as a visiting professor to initiate Asian American literature classes there. In 1991, I held an endowed chair at Trinity College in Hartford and was offered a tenured position and the directorship of the new Asian American Studies Program at the University of Wisconsin, Madison, the first in the midwest. I've received invitations to lecture internationally by such institutions as the Gorky Institute of World Literature in Moscow, Academia Sinica in Taiwan, Keio University in Tokyo, the Autonoma in Madrid, and University of Navarre in Pamplona. I'm consulted when universities wish to start Asian American Studies programs and have traveled to Utah, Illinois, Pennsylvania, and Ohio, among other places. Working to infuse multicultural literature into the American literary canon, I've co-edited seven books, including the *Heath Anthology of American Literature* and *Imagining America: Stories from the Promised Land.* To my surprise and great delight, others apparently do wish to travel down the trail a few of us have blazed.

However, as physicists tell us, every action has its reaction. When I'd finally found the perfect position for me, straddling my two worlds (professor in the English Department and director of the Asian American Studies program at the University of Wisconsin, Madison), I was alarmed to learn in my first year that my new university was threatened with budgetary cuts. In order to make informed decisions, the dean asked all chairs and directors to draft a "strategic plan" spelling out our present activities and our vision of the future. He then appointed a faculty committee to evaluate these reports and make recommendations to him. To my dismay, the faculty committee advised the dean to cut the NIUs (new instructional units)—interdisciplinary programs like Environmental Studies, Women's Studies, and all the individual Ethnic Studies programs, which the report claimed "threatened traditional departments by wanting to grow." In a time of shrinking resources, they reasoned, these NIUs should not be tolerated. The report made us sound like a cancer growing at the expense of the legitimate body. I felt as though I were nine years old again being labeled "illegal alien." Fortunately, the dean was more enlightened than his faculty committee and did not follow its recommendations.

And so my life has been a series of "versals" and reversals, a zigzagging road with turns that have advanced my progress and detours that have set me back. Some paths have been thrust on me: where I was born, who my parents would be, coming to America. Others, like pursuing Asian American literature, I've chosen to go down, bushwhacking all the way, not knowing if I would reach any destination but blazing that particular route because I had to. The longer I live, the more I see the aptness of Homer's metaphor of life: the gods on Olympus have two vials, one filled with good fortune, one with misfortune. They pour from one vial for a while and down rains good fortune. Then they decide that's enough of that and pour from the vile vial for a change. What can we mortals do but endure whatever befalls?

Women Who've Had Breast Cancer—it's not a group I would have chosen to join had I been given a choice. But of course, I hadn't. The wheel of fortune moved inexorably and on July 15, 1995 singled me out: I discovered a lump in my left breast, which, after many lengthy and painful tests, revealed infiltrating lobular carcinoma in the left breast and ductal carcinoma in situ in the right. In short, as the surgeon put it, "Cancer is busily at work in both your breasts, and we need to operate immediately."

The dreaded C word, when applied for the first time to oneself, is horrific. It feels like a death sentence for a crime one hasn't committed. "Oncologist," "lumpectomy," "chemotherapy," "hair loss," "mastectomy," and "radiation"—this entire vocabulary associated with disfigurement and death I didn't wish to claim; to put a "my" in front of any of these scorching, untouchable terms was initially unthinkable. I was incredulous: This can't be happening. It's a nightmare! Let me wake up! Why me? What have I done to deserve this? I shed rivers of tears, keeping them out of sight of my children but needing and gratefully receiving hugs and comfort from my husband. Once, in the shower, realizing that I was alone in the house, I permitted myself to release a primal scream—an expression of anguish at my unjust fate—and was pleased to discover an immediate sense of relief. Thereafter, I indulged in this secret luxury whenever the opportunity arose.

I searched for an explanation, needing a logical reason to restore sense and order to the world. What are the facts? What are the high-risk factors? Why is it I had hardly any of these factors and yet came down with the disease? What are my chances for survival? What options do I have? I tackled the disease like a research project and began to read everything I could find on the subject. The hospital distributed pamphlets; friends gave or loaned me books:

Bill Moyers's *Healing and the Mind,* Anthony Santilaro's *Recalled by Life,* Norman Cousins's *Anatomy of an Illness.* At the public library, I felt oddly displaced checking out piles of books on breast cancer instead of books for the children, novels, and literary criticism. *Dr. Susan Love's Breast Book,* Bernie Siegel's *Love, Medicine and Miracles,* Michael Lerner's *Choices in Healing*—all were helpful in various ways, informative and inspirational. Most helpful of all, however, was an unexpected occurrence that was equally devastating.

Two weeks after my diagnosis, my neighbor across the street, a neurologist, was also diagnosed with breast cancer. My situation had reminded her that she needed a mammogram, and the resultant diagnosis of her own malignancy sent her and her neurologist husband into a state of shock. She later credited me with saving her life, for helping her to catch the disease early. Hearing this news, I shed even more tears for her, knowing exactly what she was going through, but at the same time, I felt pleased (and guilty) to have a companion along the road neither of us wanted to travel.

The same surgeon performed our lumpectomies and axillary dissections (removal of lymph nodes under the arm closest to the cancer site), which were scheduled within a week of each other. Afterwards, my neighbor showed me the excruciatingly painful exercises to bring full movement back into my arm. We had different oncologists but our chemotherapy schedules overlapped. We went through the trauma of losing our hair at the same time, compared our wigs, and complimented each other on our glamorous new instant hairstyles, all the while sharing an unspoken nightmare. We parted ways when she was advised to have a mastectomy while I was told I was a likely candidate for radiation. Now we're back on the same track—taking two tamoxifen pills daily for the next five years.

More than just a companion, however, as a medical doctor, my neighbor was much more knowledgeable than I and readily gave me pointers on what to ask for. And since she was a colleague as well as a patient in our HMO, she lobbied my oncologist on my behalf, reminding him to give me a bone scan before chemotherapy began, getting me Neupogen shots when my white count went alarmingly low, sharing with me her more potent antinausea drug. In fact, the difference in the treatment we were receiving alerted me to the fact that my oncologist was more concerned about saving money than about my comfort and perhaps even my health, and led me eventually to change health plans.

Having had abdominal surgery years before, I had no problem with the surgeon's cutting into both breasts: to remove the tumor in my left breast and the site of clustered calcifications in the right. Including a margin around these sites, the surgeon took out approximately one quarter of each breast as well as a pad of fatty tissue under my left arm for the axillary dissection. As the first line of defense, lymph nodes are routinely checked to see if the cancer has spread. The lower the number of cancerous lymph nodes, the better the prognosis. In my case, one lymph node out of eleven was positive (my neighbor had zero out of ten) which meant that the spreading had begun but had not gotten too far. If all went well, the chemotherapy would take care of the wandering breast cancer cells before they set up colonies in the lungs, liver, or bones.

But chemotherapy was altogether another matter. It terrified me. Fortunately or unfortunately, I had six weeks to think about it. I'd always prided myself on putting only healthy things into my body—lots of fresh fruits and vegetables. I had never smoked, was too old for the drug scene (and wouldn't have gotten involved anyway), and rarely drank alcoholic beverages. And now the oncologist wanted me to take drugs so potent that nurses dispensing them had to wear rubber gloves, for if the chemicals should spill onto their bare skin, they would be burned. These skin-burning chemicals—Cytoxan and Adriamycin—the oncologist was proposing to inject into my bloodstream to travel throughout my body, to hunt down cancer cells. Normal cells would be destroyed as well, of course, and an overdose of Adriamycin could damage the heart muscle, he informed me. My white blood count would drop and my immune system would be so weakened that I could catch something else and die of that. By law, he was required to inform me of all the possible complications, which of course only increased my fear.

I couldn't help remembering Lynn Kellerman, once our department secretary who later became an instructor in the English Department at Livingston College. About fifteen years ago, she was suddenly stricken with uterine cancer. Lynn had chemotherapy for many months, was in remission for a year, and then the cancer recurred. Deciding that the treatment was worse than the disease, and concerned about the quality of life left to her, she refused additional chemotherapy, wasted away before our eyes, and died...at age thirty-one. We were all stunned. The cars in her funeral cortege extended for miles.

If Lynn had chosen the disease over the treatment, then chemotherapy had to be horrendous. I continued to read and to talk with friends. I learned that there are many theories but few confirmed facts, that different treatments have worked for different women. The standard treatment, which boils down to "slash, poison, and burn," began to appear extremely harsh and fundamentally misguided. Based on a principle of war, it assumes that cancer is an alien invader and that a scorched-earth policy is the best way to deal with it. Alternative treatments are based on the philosophy that the body is one whole unit and that cancer is a part of the body presently out of control, not a foreign element. If we build up the body's own immune system, it will regulate itself. Of course, the big question is how to build up the immune system so that it will be most effective against cancer. This way of thinking made a great deal more sense to me, but it was very new in the Western world and few medical centers offered it.

I began to wonder whether it had been best after all that my mother had brought me to the United States from China at age six. If my family had settled in England, I could have had an ovariectomy rather than chemotherapy; surgery seems cleaner than chemicals, and if the cancer is estrogen-fed, then it makes sense to stop the supply of estrogen. Or, if we had stayed in China, I could have seen the chi gong master that Zhen Fu Wu, a visiting scholar from Beijing, told me about. Apparently, a woman with breast cancer came all the way from England to consult Professor Zhen's chi gong master in Beijing, who gave the English woman a simple exercise to stimulate her *chi* or life energy. Professor Zhen showed me the exercise. Standing with her feet a shoulder's width apart, she slowly raised her arms out to the side, palms up, and up above her head imagining that she was gathering all the dew of the morning. Nearly closing the circle made by her arms, she imagined dropping all the gathered dew through a hole at the top of her head into the core of her body. Then very slowly, she lowered her arms, palms down, in front of her face, down past her chest, all the while envisioning the cancer cells being washed away by the shower of dew as her hands, parallel to the floor, passed down the front of her body and finally came to rest, perpendicular to the floor, at her sides. She held this position for a few moments, as though allowing the dew to fall down through her feet into the floor before starting the process again. She urged me to do this exercise for at least half an hour a day, the more frequently the better, and reported that the Englishwoman practiced this exercise several hours a day for a year with no other treatment, and her cancer disappeared.

Perhaps, if I had not left China, I might never have gotten breast cancer. Studies showed that Asian women living in Asia rarely have breast cancer. But Asian women who have lived a long time in the U.S. develop cancer at the same rate as American women. It must be something in the diet, the water, the air, the lifestyle, although my oncologist says it's simply a function of being a woman and growing older.

Dr. Santilaro in his book, *Recalled by Life,* tells of a cure effected by a macrobiotic diet of brown rice, vegetables, and miso soup.

There are claims for grass sprouts, shark cartilage, kombucha or kvass, the Essiac formula—special foods with alleged curative powers. A friend had an aunt who traveled from Florida to Toronto to see a cancer specialist who staved off her uterine cancer with a special drug and massive doses of vitamin C. Maxine Hong Kingston invited me to go to the Pine Street Clinic in California where someone she knew meditated several hours a day for a year and was now fine. The array of alternative possibilities became overwhelming.

Finally, I made a decision on a practical basis: my pocketbook. Alternative treatments would have to be paid for out of pocket while standard treatments were covered by my health insurance. As the sole support for my family of four, I couldn't afford to be extravagant or experimental. Furthermore, individual success stories did not prove anything. These were the stories of survivors; those who had died could not tell us, "Don't go this route. It doesn't work." Conventional treatment had undergone scientific tests, which seemed to demonstrate a certain amount of effectiveness. The survival rate seemed determined by how early one caught the disease. The earlier the stage, the smaller the tumor, the fewer affected lymph nodes, the better the survival rate. That unconventional or Eastern methods had not undergone Western scientific tests was no proof that they didn't work but, for me, in Madison, Wisconsin, they would be inconvenient, expensive, and risky. I felt trapped, forced by circumstances to take a path I didn't like.

With a heavy heart and tremendous fear, I set a date, appeared on time, sat down in what I imagined to be an execution chair, and with tears streaming allowed the nurse to inject the two vials of vile chemicals into a vein in my wrist. After the terror I'd built up, I was surprised that I was able to walk out of the hospital afterwards. An hour later the nausea hit, and every hour thereafter for three days, I was vomiting and retching. Hoping to save money, the doctor had prescribed Compazine for the nausea, an old drug that cost $1 a tablet, instead of Zofran, a new drug costing $19 a pill. When I was unable to hold down any food or drink for three days, he finally suggested that I come to the hospital for intravenous hydration. Two liters later, I was still nauseous and needed to be kept overnight. The doctor's effort to save money resulted only in our having to spend even more—to say nothing of my suffering.

Although the oncologist advised me to stop working during the chemotherapy treatments, I'd sought out and spoken with women who had continued to work the entire time they were receiving the same two chemicals I would be receiving, and I'd also read that chemotherapy was not as debilitating as it had been, for certain studies had shown that smaller and fewer doses were equally effective. So I decided to continue to work: to meet my classes and to administer the small Asian American Studies Program. However, not knowing in advance how my body would respond, I wanted to be prepared in case I was totally debilitated. My department rallied to my assistance in a most heartwarming way. The chair sent a copy of my syllabus to all members of the department, asking for volunteers to be prepared to teach one text in the course in the event of my inability to do so. Within a week, every text on my syllabus had been taken, and for certain texts there were even multiple volunteers. My mind was at rest on this score, and I was deeply touched by this evidence of my colleagues' support.

As word went around, many expressed concern and love through bouquets (more flowers than I'd had at my two weddings combined), cards, letters, long distance and international phone calls. My sister-in-law, her Japanese husband, and three children folded one thousand paper cranes and mailed them in a large carton from Great Falls, Virginia. I had no idea that so many people cared. My falling ill so suddenly and so seriously probably reminded them how precarious a hold on life we each have, how each of us lives with Damocles' sword hanging by a thread over our heads.

Since my classes met on Tuesdays and Thursdays, I scheduled chemotherapy injections for Thursday afternoons, which allowed me four days to recover. I spent most of those four days in bed but was able to read sufficiently to be prepared for class on Tuesday. My protocol called for a total of four injections of Adriamycin and Cytoxan to be given at three-week intervals, but my white blood count was generally so low that the next injection was nearly always delayed. Between injections, despite the low white count and weakness, I was able to be up and about and to lead what seemed on the surface to be a fairly normal life.

Two things, however, were very abnormal. First, I had to have injections of Neupogen every night for two weeks after chemotherapy. I was shocked to learn that the cost of this drug to elevate the white blood count depressed by chemotherapy was $1,000 for a two-week supply. It seemed all too clear to me that drug companies were making a fortune, but since I had decided to put my life in the hands of the "experts" (although I questioned their reasoning), I went along with the program. Learning to stab myself in the leg never became easy or routine. Each night I approached the moment with enormous dread, so that most times my husband took over the onerous chore. While my eleven-year-old daughter clutched my hand, chanting, "It's keeping you out of the hospital. It's keeping you out of the hospital," my husband would make the jab, hoping to catch me unawares and trying not to hit a vein, which would then leave me black and blue for weeks.

The other difficult aspect was losing my hair. Two weeks after the first chemotherapy injection, I'd run my fingers through my hair and find twenty or thirty strands between each finger. I sat in front of the wastebasket combing my hair with my fingers, releasing them from their roots, tears streaming down my cheeks. Hair, after all, is a person's glory, a natural crown setting off one's facial features. I did not like the prospect of being bald—even if certain rock stars, as my husband informed me, thought baldness cool and had shaved their heads. They had a choice. One early October morning, I went into the nature conservancy across the street from our house, found myself a spot to sit undisturbed, and "seeded" the woods with my hair. Earth to earth, I thought, ashes to ashes. The leaves were turning gold and scarlet, the sun was warm, and no one intruded on my solitude and my grieving. I sat there quietly, and it soon became a peaceful moment of acceptance of what could not be helped.

What could be helped, however, was to turn this unwanted necessity into an opportunity. Since I couldn't have my own hair, I would have whatever hair I wanted. When I discovered a wholesale beauty supply store that sold wigs to cancer patients at cost—$25—I decided to buy several to change around in, depending on my mood. I had a total of three wigs. The first, my serious professional wig, cost over $100 at J. C. Penney's before I discovered the wholesale store. A sixties bob, straight and black with bangs, it was as close to my own hair as I could find. The other two, cheaper and much more fun, came from the discount store. The wig I called Cher was also black but had loose curls falling halfway down my back. My favorite, Annie, was short, curly and...strawberry blond. As a child, like Toni Morrison's Pecola Breedlove, I'd longed to be a blond; as an adult, I recognized such longings as self-rejection and intellectually rejected them. But as a cancer patient, I wanted to pamper myself and satisfy an irrational craving. I didn't care if I was being politically incorrect. Surprisingly, this curly blond wig did not look as strange with my Chinese features and skin tone as I'd expected when first trying it on as a lark. I looked, as Han Suyin put it, "not bad." Certain clothes in the brown tones even looked better with strawberry blond hair. And best of all, I could clasp my hands together, look up at the ceiling, and sing Li'l Orphan Annie's so-appropriate song, "Tomorrow, tomorrow, I love ya, tomorrow./You're only a day away."

I survived the four months of chemotherapy needing colleague coverage for only two classes, one of those for bronchitis. Then came another crossroad requiring a decision: mastectomy or radiation? The surgeon urged double mastectomy, cleaner and worry-free. The radiologist advised five weeks of daily radiation with an extra week of an electron boost. The prospect of losing both breasts, small as mine were, caused me extreme distress; I couldn't see it as anything other than an amputation. Two pieces of art I saw in a Bill Moyers's *Healing and the Mind* caused me to burst into tears. *Cradling Her Sorrow* (1989) by Nancy Fried was the startling bust of a headless woman cradling her head in her arms. In place of her right breast was a scar. George Tooker's *Farewell*, entirely in shades of pale blue, showed a small female figure overwhelmed by the long square corridor of squares she was walking down; she stood at the cross formed by powerful diagonal lines of perspective. These pieces, which captured the anguish of mutilation and death, spoke eloquently to me and for me on a deep intuitive level. I was in a quandary, forced once more to make a choice between two options, neither of which I liked.

I asked the three male doctors—surgeon, oncologist, and radiologist—to confer and come up with one recommendation. They were the experts; I would trust their joint decision. Finally, the surgeon was persuaded by the others that radiation was the way to go, that the side effects were minimal—only sunburn and chafing, and that I could always come back to him if I had a recurrence. Despite my joy at keeping my breasts, I next had to overcome the fear of radiation. In my head swarmed images of the survivors of Hiroshima and Nagasaki—radiation burned and destroyed in horrible ways. My sister, an emergency room physician, said that radiated flesh never healed properly afterwards. Again, it was speaking with women who had gone through the treatment that gave me the courage to accept it for myself.

In March, the radiation came to an end and now that the "sunburn" has peeled away and my energy has returned, I'm feeling back to normal. There are many days I don't think about breast cancer at all. Life goes on as before, and I assume it will continue. Of course, there is always the possibility of recurrence, that I'll be derailed again. I've met a woman who was clear for ten years and then the boom fell again. As soldiers face death on the battlefield, cancer patients must all wrestle with the possibility of our own deaths. Once more, I've had no choice, but I have faced my mortality and accepted it. As the Vietnamese Zen master Thich Nhat Hanh has written: "We see that life and death are but two faces of Life and that without both, Life is not possible, just as two sides of a coin are needed for the coin to exist."[2]

However, *being* both sides of the coin simultaneously is an extremely difficult condition. Threatened by a cancer within my own body, I've fought both to control and to eliminate it by taking two different routes. In one way, I see the disease as a spiritual wake-up call, my body and soul's rebellion against being taken for granted, being so long ignored in my obsessive-compulsive intellectual striving for economic survival and academic success. At a cellular level, my body—the temple of my soul—is demanding respectful attention and gentle nurturing. I'm being reminded to look within, to reorder and balance my priorities. Yet, I've also taken the standard route of "slash, poison, and burn" to destroy the malignant cells that, if left unchecked, would sabotage the entire body, for they mean me no good.

My work and my identity have also placed me in two impossible positions at once. Working to expand the literary canon by advocating inclusion of ethnic American literature, especially Asian American, I have been perceived by some in the academy as a cancer seeking to grow at the expense of the rest of the traditional academic body. But is Asian American literature really an alien invader threatening the ivory tower? If I teach students to read Maxine Hong Kingston and David Henry Hwang, does it automatically follow that Shakespeare will not be taught and that Western Civilization as we've known it will die? Perhaps that part of Western Civilization that is imbued with unquestioned imperialist, sexist, and racist assumptions should die or at least be transformed into a truly equitable, inclusive, less hegemonic entity.

As an Asian American woman I stand between the worlds of white and black. When I join groups working for solidarity and coalition among peoples of color, I sense that some African

Americans resent my presence; for them, Asian Americans have already made it and are only taking up valuable resources. I can see their point and do not disagree that among Asians only Southeast Asians are now designated "targeted minorities" eligible for federal assistance. Yet, if Asian American high school students study hard and earn the grades to gain them admission into the nation's top-ranking universities, is it really fair that they be excluded for taking up too many places at the expense of other students in this country? On the other hand, how can we not educate all the members of our society? No one should be designated a cancer destined for destruction.

How can one survive being both the cancer and the body politic?

I certainly don't have the answers. I just know that I must live with contradictions. Finally, and paradoxically, being forced to face my death, I have come to appreciate how full and satisfying my life actually is. With a loving and beloved husband and two healthy children, a career I thoroughly enjoy, books with my name on their spines, visits to all corners of the globe, I've been unusually privileged and blessed. In the large scheme of things, my problems have been relatively few, and I've been fortunate to see my handicaps transformed into strengths. If my time were up now, I could go— gently, into that good night, with grace and with gratitude.

Notes

[1] "Incident" by Countee Cullen from Abraham Chapman, ed., *Black Voices: An Anthology of Afro-American Literature* (New York: Mentor Books, 1968), pp. 384-385.

Incident

Once riding in old Baltimore,
    Heart-filled, head-filled with glee,
I saw a Baltimorean
    Keep looking straight at me.

Now I was eight and very small,
And he was no whit bigger,
And so I smiled, but he poked out
His tongue and called me, "Nigger."

I saw the whole of Baltimore
From May until December:
Of all the things that happened there
That's all that I remember.

[2] Thich Nhat Hanh, *The Miracle of Mindfulness: A Manual on Meditation,* trans. Mobi Ho (Boston: Beacon Press, 1987), p. 51.

Hilda Raz

❧

Getting Well

If I get well… I can take a walk in the snow and eat a red apple.
—Anne Truitt, Turn

You gave me four fair hairs
from your head, locked in the pages
you left Monday morning in my mailbox,
a sign of the passion of your reading.

You would have me know how to write
an essay, commissioned, on the stuff of my life
on this model, Truitt's, or any other
we might find together, the pleasure

of our reading in concert as colleagues
hiding our camaraderie in health,
your sure recovery from the disease
I'm sure will take me off.

So I touch the binding, unsure
of what you mean to say. Work
can keep us alive to the world?
Writing down some truth will help?

What I know today has something
to do with your hair, caught
in a book's pages. Fair
you stand up in the world

to walk. Fair, you sit down
in the sun to read, your head
bent down to eat an apple. Here,
you draw in the breath of the air
and breathe it out so we can write.

Claudia MonPere McIsaac

❧

Flowers, Bones

ON TOP OF A SNOW-COVERED MOUNTAIN, MY mother holds an ice-axe, a rope slung around her shoulder. She is the single spot of color in a rugged landscape where nothing but a few stunted bushes survive.

Mother didn't have hobbies the way other people do. Whatever she was doing, she threw herself into it with an intensity and drive for perfection: cross-country skiing, backpacking, opera, gardening, photography, art history, interior design, ceramics, painting.

In the years following her death from breast cancer, I've tried to make sense out of my mother's life. She documented events with remarkable precision, leaving behind: thirteen photo albums, four scrapbooks from high school and college, eight notebooks containing everything from lists of her imperfections and goals for improvement to quotations from the Bible and literary works, a series of travel logs, six art journals with ideas and sketches for her art projects.

And two maroon record books. In these books my mother records her thoughts during my childhood when she suffered from serious depression:

—A new year and how I hope to be well again. There are times when I think I will never make it.

—Right now I'm cowering in my room waiting for Dr. D to get me admitted to the hospital. I can't sleep. I weigh 94 pounds.

—Horrible day. I took out the seconal pills and counted them, rolled
   them between my fingers. No hysteria, just quiet agony.

My mother's hospitalizations usually resulted from terrible fits
of hysteria and depression, sometimes combined with drinking, or
complete failure to sleep or eat for days at a time. Her journal is
filled with vivid descriptions of nightmarish dreams: her children
dead or dying, her family abandoning her, grotesque monsters
imprisoning her. "I have never been loved," she writes.

But the desperate mother of my youth was not the same woman
as the mother who died at age fifty-four. She bore the same name
and, until her last weeks, looked the same although older: creamy
skin peppered with freckles, a delicate frame with long graceful
legs, intense green eyes. But this older woman had a confidence
and joy that had eluded her in her younger years.

It had come late in life, this new self. A new therapist, her six
children's movement into adulthood, her decision to return to college and study art—these things and others came together to shape
her into someone quite different from the mother I knew when I
was a child.

I can't remember a time when I didn't worry about her. I'd open
the door carefully when I returned from school, not sure what I'd
find. She might be gardening or rearranging furniture. Or. The
house might be dark, my brothers and sisters sobbing in their
rooms, my mother's door locked. I'd put my ear to her door, listening. Was she sleeping? Weeping? Had she hurt herself?

And the rages. I have hazy memories of her waving knives
around in the kitchen, her face looking like a wounded animal's as
she yells. She hates us, we hate her, no one cares whether she lives
or dies, she is nothing. A child can take a tiny incident and work
it into something monstrous over the years, use memory as clay to
shape and pummel so that what finally stays in a brain bears little
resemblance to the thing as it happened. As an adult I figured my
overactive imagination had conjured up the image: my mother

turning on the kitchen lights, the room redolent with the smell of burnt roast. Mother is screaming, and we children are crying and holding each other. She grabs a butcher knife. I spread my arms around me like wings, shielding my younger siblings. The blade gleams in the kitchen's fluorescent light, dances through the air, more a display of fury in motion than a real threat—too far away from us, really, to hurt anyone. We watch, unblinking, as it slashes the smoky air.

When I discovered my mother's journals, I realized the image was real. After her death, her many notebooks were put away. Five years later, sorting through old boxes, I was stunned to uncover page after page documenting pieces of her life. I'd known about the art journals. But the rest I'd never seen before. I read it all. And as I hold the crumbling pages of *Campus Classroom Chatter*, the high school newspaper column she wrote; as I finger the dust from an old corsage; as I weep at the blackness that swallowed her for many years, documented so clearly in her journals; as I rejoice at the sketches and tiny paintings in her art notebooks, I realize what a gift she left. And I try to put the pieces together. I try to understand my mother in a way I did not understand her while she lived.

When Mother told me she had breast cancer, she spoke lightly, as if she were referring to a wart that needed removing. The doctor had caught the cancer early. The double mastectomy was a simple procedure. She'd be miffed if I missed my friend's wedding for such a thing. (To this day I do not forgive myself for sitting in the warm Los Angeles sun eating shrimp while my mother had her breasts removed.)

Although the cancer had invaded a few lymph nodes, her doctors were optimistic about a full recovery. Radiation and chemotherapy became a part of Mother's life, but they didn't take over. She painted, gardened, attended Mass, read—she continued doing the things she loved. My youngest brother was out of the country, and he remembers the huge care packages Mother sent him at that time—baskets that spewed forth caramels, cookies, peanut brittle, fudge. Only days after the surgery, my mother was shopping for a dress to wear to my sister Julie's upcoming wedding, annoyed at how her external I.V. made it hard to change in the dressing room. I went with her a few times for her radiation treatment, and it was clear from her jokes with the technicians that she refused to think of herself as a cancer victim.

In fact, her oncologist's sober and sometimes cold demeanor irritated her. When my mother lost her hair, she found her wig itchy and hot and sometimes didn't wear it. Hearing this, her oncologist admonished her about making others uncomfortable seeing a bald woman. One day when she waited in the examining room, she saw him walking down the hall. She poked her head out of the room and called his name, doffing her wig as if it were a hat. Determined to make him smile, once in the hospital she hid her face behind a newspaper, and when he came up to her bed, swept the paper aside to reveal her face in Groucho Marx attire, complete with glasses, big nose, and mustache.

Before the cancer, my mother moved with a sizzle. Living in Fresno so close to the mountains, I spent my childhood summers backpacking with my family in the Sierra Nevadas. Mother was passionate about the mountains. In her less severe depressions, a trip to the Sierras could bring a lilt to her voice in a way nothing else could. Exhausted from a long hike to our campsite, the rest of us would collapse on the ground while my mother tore off her dusty clothes and plunged into an icy lake. While we relaxed with a book or played cards later in the day, she could be seen scrambling across boulder fields, putting together driftwood sculptures, photographing mushrooms clinging to a fallen pine. She was a paradox—a study in both motion and fragility.

The chemotherapy slowed her down to the kind of pace most of us live by.

I was stunned at how my mother responded when she learned she had cancer, at how quickly she snapped back to her normal routine after a few days of crying. At how she laughed off the loss of two breasts: "They were so small anyway. There's not much to miss." She displayed a painterly curiosity and in her art journal constructed what she called a mastectomy palette—yellow, red-violet, blue green, purple. Fascinated by the crablike shape of cancer cells, she had my brother, a doctor, draw them so she could incorporate them into a painting project.

With the flush of guilt from missing her surgery still strong within me, I worried. I read everything I could find about breast cancer. I cut out articles on experimental treatments. I think I drove my physician father, my physician brother, and my sister, Julie, who is a nurse, crazy with questions. I remember the big pile of books on breast cancer and chemotherapy that I got for my mother. She thanked me politely and put them on her nightstand. A spy, I peeked at the books over the following months to see if they were being read. But never a bookmark or note in the margin. After a while, they disappeared.

I was distressed by what I interpreted as my mother's passivity in the face of such a serious illness. How in the world, I wondered, could a person have cancer and not want to learn about it? But I have learned that there is no universal response to illness. Mother wanted to keep the cancer peripheral to her life. She had no interest in a cancer support group, and when an old friend who now had breast cancer contacted her, she was disappointed that all they discussed was cancer. She'd had many bleak years in her past, times when she crawled into her head and was so conscious of the pain that she felt raw, skinned. Those days were over. Having worked so long to create a healthy mind and spirit, she wasn't about to dwell on her body's betrayal.

Although her journals at this time focus primarily on her art, she weaves in short references to cancer, comments couched mostly in humor and optimism:

—Cancer victim—no way!

—I had a cancer dream last night. I met a man who said that when he
had chemotherapy his arms were burned by the radiation. I danced
with him, however, and he seemed to use his arms in a normal manner. His feet were not so great, however!

—It's not everyone who is lucky enough to be given a second chance
in life! This time around I'll do it right!

Her breasts were gone. Her hair fell out in dry tufts. She was
tired and nauseated from the chemotherapy. She was brave, so
brave, and I was surprised and moved by her courage. Although
I lived three hours away, we spoke on the phone often. And
when we did, it wasn't about cancer or pain or fear. It was about
my young daughter or my teaching. Or painting projects she
was working on. Or about the red flowers she saw blooming by
the road.

But while she didn't worry in front of her children, comments
crept into her art journal that weren't so stoic: "I think phase 1 of
this terrible thing is over and I won't always try being so cheerful
and saying it was a good thing that happened to me. I won't play
the Polly Anna game quite so much any more." And a few weeks
later: "Dead is dead is dead."

Reading my mother's journals after her death, I sensed that in
my childhood, my siblings and I were a ghost family to her, like
the San Joaquin Valley tulle fog that swirled around knotted fig
trees, vanished the orchards in damp white silence.

It was her childhood family that seemed carved into her heart
and bones. We lived close to her parents when I was growing up, a
tiny pasture between us. My mother writes, "My father's tractor
going back and forth, the sheep bleating, their dog barking, their
voices talking in the yard—these are things which can set me into
a fury."

My grandmother was obsessed with social propriety—garden parties, bridge games, charity events. She was highly critical of my mother as she was growing up and forbade any show of strong emotion. My grandfather treated my mother with a combination of scorn and neglect, mocking her for her allergies, refusing to give up his pet poodles that sent her into fits of wheezing, killing raccoons and possums in front of her and laughing at her fear.

My mother was nine or ten when she began banging her head against the wall. Slowly, rhythmically, then faster and faster, a metronome that could almost keep time to her mother's fingers playing ragtime on the piano or the strains from her father's mandolin.

Growing up with a mother who for many years darted in and out of our lives like a lilac shadow, we six children had strong feelings about her, feelings tinged with sorrow, anger, guilt—and a deep, abiding love. My father was patient and loving, earnest in his explanations that we weren't to blame for my mother's unhappiness. And in her good periods, Mother was affectionate, humorous, enthusiastic, protective. I can still smell the musty odor of my grandparents' closet where I hid as a child because of some sick trick my grandfather played on me with a bloody finger. My mother screamed at him, the veins on her thin neck bulging.

I never stopped loving my mother. Yet mixed in with that love was a sadness that she'd been so unavailable when I was a child. Then as she began healing, I was older, away from home, caught up in my own life. I remember the jealousy I felt as an adult, shopping with my mother and youngest sister, Amy, for a trip my sister was going to take. My mother's concern that my sister be warm enough and that she have comfortable shoes for walking was touching. But I wanted to snatch some of that nurturing and cram it into my pre-teen years when I wore unfashionable clothes and tried to be a little mother to my younger siblings.

In the last few years before her cancer, however, my mother and I had spent some wonderful times together—hiking in Yosemite, poking around antique shops, photographing old graveyards. I have a photograph of her lying on top of a grave marker, clutching a bouquet of wildflowers, eyes closed, grinning.

As Mother's chemotherapy and radiation progressed, I couldn't let go of the thought that she'd been in my life for a few years but would vanish again. This time forever.

Perhaps the strongest passion in my mother's life at the time she was diagnosed with cancer was her art. Through the fatigue and nausea, she worked on a range of projects—an oil painting of me nursing my daughter, a sketch of four Hmong women, a collage of children's war toys, a Hiroshima watercolor. About a year before her surgery, she'd developed a profound interest in the archeological ruins of the Southwest, particularly the Anasazi Indians and their rock art. Her art journals of this time include notes on hunting magic, astronomical readings, fertility rites, clan symbols. When her nausea was particularly bad and the smell of paints made her sick, she worked in other mediums. She and my father took a trip to the Southwest where they climbed in caves, photographing petroglyphs of bighorn sheep and primitive human figures. She developed a technique in which she repro- duced her color photos on a copy machine and then manipulated the images with Prismacolor pencil, layering the surfaces with rich, intense colors.

My mother was born with an artist's eye. It's apparent in her early charcoal sketches. Just a girl, she caught the flare of a horse's nostrils, the lacy breath of a willow. She attended college, but her parents didn't want her to study art. After two years, she got mar- ried and had children. The six of us came quickly and the charcoal and paints were moved to the back of a closet.

Her home became her obsession as she prowled thrift shops and garage sales for interesting furniture, sewed pillows and tablecloths, purchased inexpensive prints that looked stunning when she framed them. Easter brought hand-painted eggs hanging from a branch she'd driven to the foothills to find, then dyed white. Christmas meant handmade wreaths, elaborate nativity scenes. When I was seven, happiest playing with my Barbie and Ken dolls, my mother sewed lush hooded gowns for them, placing them in a manger with a baby doll and some ceramic sheep and cows. At night, I'd crawl out of bed to stroke the thick velvet of Ken's purple robe, Barbie's blue cape.

As I grew older, I'd wonder about these sewing and craft tasks that she set for herself. They gave her pleasure but also produced enormous tension. If guests for the Christmas Eve open house would be arriving soon and the floral display she'd been working on wasn't quite right, she'd crumble and the evening might be ruined. For God's sake, I'd angrily think, why didn't she just order the flowers? Why put this kind of pressure on herself? But I think now that perhaps these were all substitutes for the painting that was impossible with six young children, a socially acceptable way in the fifties and sixties for a woman to channel her artistic sensibilities.

A few years before my mother got cancer, she went back to college to study art. She was terrified in those early classes, felt inadequate, worried about how her teachers and fellow students would judge her. She began keeping an art journal and wrote that "since I'm so nervous my friend Carol suggested I spill catsup on the first page and thus make a beginning." The first page, titled *Fantasy Map: A Study in Catsup, Mustard, and Ink,* is an artistic rendering of an imaginary map with the address of every place she's lived. The entire map is cradled in mountains and sun, mermaids lolling in the sea.

Reading these art journals, one can see the progress from a talented but timid novice obsessed with others' approval to a confident artist. Worried she lacked ideas for composition, my mother at first copied other paintings or composed lovely yet very traditional oil landscapes. But as she visited countless galleries and museums and took class after class, she experimented with color and shape. Her oils became more abstract, the subjects often satiric or fanciful—a line of empty voting booths, the American flag at the side; an old door covered with graffiti; a vine-covered birdbath where pruning shears are turning into birds. She joined a gallery and her work began to sell. I loved it all. In my sister's kitchen hangs a favorite of mine—a Dove detergent bottle that my mother engineered to look like an exaggerated version of a shapely, perky housewife—Brillo pad for hair, face slathered in makeup, exaggerated breasts, tiny mops for hands. Sort of a Barbie Becomes a Detergent Bottle.

My mother drew and wrote in her art journals until shortly before she died. Remarkable documents, these journals are filled with ideas for paintings and ceramics, preliminary sketches, musings on artists who were influencing her, inspirational quotes from poets and philosophers, reflections on her dreams. About a year before she died, she began to compose haiku and these, too, are included. Lovely nature haiku and a series of opening lines for cancer haiku that she began but put aside: "If not me, who then?" "I long for routine," "Shhhhh . . . cancer at work."

*   *   *

We had a second wedding in the family. My sister, Amy, was married in August in the red boil of summer. Mother's chemotherapy had ended eight months earlier and she was happy and energetic as she helped plan the wedding in Fresno. The colors Amy had chosen, white and green, suggested new life, innocence, renewal.

A few days after the wedding we learned Mother's cancer had returned, this time invading her bones.

She dove into living with a fury, her fingers whirring in her garden, at her easel. She wasn't able to go to the opera that fall, a bitter disappointment. She loved the Bay Area, and it had been her special treat to herself for the last few years, that trip on the bus to the spectacle of the San Francisco Opera. Mother begged me to take her tickets and be especially nice to the elderly woman who sat next to her, with whom she'd struck up a friendship. The woman had a heart problem and my mother was worried about her.

Mother had always wished someone in our family would share her passion for opera. I can remember dozing through three or four operas with her over the years until one evening she took me to *The Flying Dutchman* where, much to her delight, I was won over by the tattered sails and ghastly blood light and the singing that seemed to rip open the throats of the people on stage.

And it was Wagner that she watched that fall as she began another round of chemo. Sitting in front of the television, she lost herself in the music's thunder, a metal bowl in her lap as she vomited.

In spite of the cancer's metastasis, my mother's interest in pre-Columbian art continued to grow. In the middle of this second round of chemotherapy, she and my father decided to go to Mexico. Her oncologist had her on oral medication and cautioned her about the risk of serious infection because her immune system was so weak. It was clearly a risky trip but one she'd wanted to make for a long time. She was in pain, but it was kept under control with medication. My father remembers her energy during those three weeks. After viewing museums in Mexico City and ruins in the Yucatan, she pored over guidebooks and maps, planning outings to more obscure sights. They drove and drove, often the only car on a bumpy road with jungle on either side. When they arrived at a ruin, she'd bound around sketching and taking photos. She walked up the crumbling steps of pyramids, wove through dark passages and narrow wet stairways, climbed down into excavated graves, bottles of pills rattling in her backpack.

Mother returned from the trip to Mexico with renewed optimism. I hovered at the fringes, terrified she was going to die. My sister, Julie, a nurse, knew more than I. I think this knowledge pressed inside her, an iron cage that I tried to pry open but that remained clamped shut. She wanted to spend time with my mother but didn't want to talk odds. My other sister, Amy, believed always that my mother would recover. Loving them both fiercely, I found the silence of one and the Pollyanna attitude of the other as maddening as they must have found my endless pecking for grains of truth, probabilities, options.

We spend my mother's last Christmas at the coast. All of my brothers and sisters and our families are there, crammed into a rental house. The grandchildren toddle around putting baskets on their heads, rolling oranges on the kitchen floor. We roast a huge turkey with stuffing and sweet potatoes. My mother eats rice and banana because she is so nauseated from the chemo. She is tired and in pain. But she also has spunk. "Let's go outside and take some photographs," she tells me and my sisters.

We grab our cameras, walk into the foggy morning, and smell the salt air. We walk to a nearby marsh where there are egrets, ducks, Canada geese. In a mass of green and white by the water, my mother finds some puma grass, the stalks taller than us, the ends light and feathery. Perfect brooms. We twist and pull, getting one for each of us. Sticking them between our legs, we gallop in bold circles. My mother takes off her wig, waves it around like a brown pom-pom. Her scalp is pinkish and shiny, mostly bald with a little fuzz. Like my daughter's head when she was a few days old. We run along the marsh and the geese run too, their wings batting the wind, their honking and our shouts swept into the fog.

Spring. For a few months there had been hope that the second round of chemotherapy and radiation would get the cancer under control. But suddenly my mother's pain worsens almost daily. She and my father spend a week at a small coastal town in Northern California. My father remembers the wildflowers blooming, lupin and poppies flaming the coastal grasses, Queen Anne's lace spilling onto the road. His birthday is that week. Mother's pain radiates throughout her body, but they walk and admire the flowers. Mother has brought along a memoir by a woman whose mother died of cancer, and she and my father take turns reading it to each other. They walk and they read. And it settles in them, that week, the knowledge that the chemotherapy has failed. They talk about dying.

New tests reveal the cancer has gone wild. Intensive radiation, expected to have a palliative effect, does nothing. One day Mother turns to answer the phone and breaks a bone. In the hospital, she is either in great pain or so heavily sedated it's difficult for her to communicate.

My five brothers and sisters and I make arrangements with work and childcare and spend as much time as we can in the hospital. I leave the Bay Area every Thursday with my toddler daughter, Angela, and stay with my mother until Monday. This goes on for about six weeks, and when I think of how much time I spent at St. Agnes Hospital, it seems strange that no sustained pattern of events comes to me.

But memory is not a line. Rather, there are discrete moments so finely etched in my mind I can smell them, taste them, see them in their sad, glorious colors.

I start to enter her hospital room, then stop, watching her from the doorway. She is wearing handsome horn-rimmed glasses. Utterly engaged in the newspaper she is reading, she doesn't see me. Her bed jacket is no frilly pink thing but a deep coffee brown with a tailored cut. I squint my eyes to block out the I.V. and for a moment believe she is in a fancy hotel waiting for room service to bring her eggs Benedict.

Another day. I bring her a funny Diane Keaton movie. Popcorn, too, forgetting she can't eat it. Mother loved popcorn, savored it during a movie, ate it kernel by kernel so that halfway through the movie her container was still full while the rest of us had only oily kernels to suck on.

We watch Diane Keaton and laugh. My mother touches the popcorn, rolls a piece between her fingers, holds a pile to her nose and breathes in the salty, buttery scent.

And another day. My father and I are helping my mother out of bed for one of her twice-daily walks around the floor. Really, it is more of a shuffle due to her pain and the fact she must walk with the I.V. rolling alongside her. Yet these walks have taken on a monumental importance for her. My father puts her slippers on. I am shocked at how yellow her toenails are, and when I worry to him later that she is getting an ingrown toenail, he just stares at me. It hurts Mother to move, but she is finally sitting at the side of the bed. Before we help her stand, my father says, "Wait a minute. I have something for you."

He hands her a small silver box and opens it. Inside is a corsage, an elegant gardenia with a sparkling silver ribbon. He pins it on her hospital gown. As they ready themselves for the slow walk down the hospital corridor, he draws her to him, asking, "My dear, will you dance the St. Agnes Shuffle with me?"

Dying. It took three days. There was a beginning, a middle, an end.

My mother told us she was going home to die. She'd been on medication to lower the dangerously high levels of calcium in her blood. She wanted to stop the medication and go home. She would slip into a coma and be dead in a matter of days.

What do you say when your mother tells you she's had enough? Enough wrenching pain. Enough needles and pills and radiation. Enough fractured bones. Enough fuzzy thought and slurred speech.

Her oncologist wanted her to begin more chemo. But he was honest about how unlikely it was that it would slow the cancer's spread. Still, he was passionate about fighting with whatever it took. It was an on-call oncologist who had seen her in the hospital before who held her hand while she cried from the pain and said, "You don't have to go on like this."

I remember standing around my mother's hospital bed with my father and brothers and sisters hearing my mother say she wanted to go home to die. I remember, after that first mad gulp for air, how quickly and compassionately they supported her decision. And I remember burying the voice within me that was shouting, "No, my God, no. Let's discuss this. What are the options? What kinds of experimental programs are available? Why can't she try more chemo and see if by some slim chance it will work? For God's sake, how can we just give up?"

I said nothing.

And for a long time, a very long time, I thought each night that maybe if I'd been more assertive, been rude, even, made a scene—somehow things might have been different. Was this egotism at its worst? Or was it the terror and grief of someone losing her mother just as she was getting to know her?

My sister Julie tells me: "I see people dying in ungodly ways. They suffer and they suffer and they suffer. Mom had a zest for life and she did not give up easily. She knew when it was time to go. Claudia, you can't let your wishes be someone else's."

Mother's return home was a quite a production. It took many trips up and down the elevator to get all the flowers, photographs, tapes, books. Two years earlier, I'd been in the hospital a long time when I was pregnant and in premature labor. I had a bizarre feeling of déjà vu now, remembering packing up all the objects that my family had sent to my hospital room to cheer me up. Except that I had returned home to be a new mother. My mother was returning home to die.

We rented a hospital bed for her bedroom. Between the king-size bed and the sleeping bags we dragged in, there was room for my father and all six of us. Except for short breaks, we pretty much lived in that room those three days. I don't want to romanticize that time. But if dying can be good, this was.

We prayed together, we talked, we read. There were young children wandering in and out. They knew only that their grandmother was very sick and they spent a great deal of time placing small toys beside her bed to make her feel better. There was music—Beethoven, Mozart, Bach, and, of course, some exquisite arias. We'd placed Mother's bed close to the window with the curtains open so she could see her garden. The begonias and fuchsias were in bloom, and purple lantana tumbled over rocks. The maple had a hummingbird feeder hanging from it, and we could watch the flicker of crimson and blue feathers.

Home health-care nurses came and went. It must have been confusing for them, entering a house to care for a dying woman, discovering her six adult children unwilling to leave her room, the husband, son, and daughter huddled over the *Physician's Desk Reference* trying to figure out what dosage of narcotics would keep her comfortable but not kill her. The morphine was on a shelf in my parents' closet. To the right was a pair of running shoes. To the left was Mother's Styrofoam wig stand. Months earlier, she'd painted a funny face on it.

Mother wasn't scared. Her faith sustained her. Her priest had spent many mornings at her bedside, and he supported her decision to go home and die. I think she was also sustained by the knowledge that although much of her life had been spent in a haze of depression, her last years had been full and good. She'd grown into her identity as an artist—the last card she sent her mother is signed, "Love, your artist daughter, Susan." But more significant than her art, I think, is that she knew she loved us and we loved her. Through many difficult years, we had all learned to treat one another with kindness and respect. And that is no small thing. I talk to my friends and hear stories of parents refusing to speak to a son or daughter for years on end; of siblings who cannot be together without a bitter eruption of old rivalries; of fights over money, property, or furniture. And I think of my mother and father, my brothers and sisters, and I know what we shared was unusual. And I know why she could die with no regrets.

*   *   *

I am outwardly calm, choosing my mother's clothes for the church service, helping to write her eulogy. At night I dream of bones, see her body splintering bit by bit till it is a mass of white shards.

While I am searching my parents' bookshelves for poems to be read at her funeral, I think, "I could write one. Not to read at the service, of course, but maybe something for my family." A full-time teaching job and motherhood have taken me far away from writing. But now I write a poem about my mother swimming in a mountain lake, the first poem I've written since college.

After my mother is cremated, I hike with my husband and father, siblings, and in-laws to a spot my mother loved high in the Sierra Nevada mountains. We clasp hands and one by one read something we've prepared. I read my poem and remember my mother telling me to write and write and let nothing get in my way. We scatter her ashes. There is a slight wind and some of the ashes fly back at us, drift toward our bodies, land at our feet on the silver-flecked granite. We laugh and we cry as we try to retrieve the dust of my mother and send it to cerulean basins below.

Like many women, I have fibrocystic breasts that are difficult to examine. When I was a teenager, I had two breast biopsies, which proved to be benign. The scars were fairly large and, undressing in gym class, I tried to hide them. I observed the change in color and shape over the years and was relieved when they finally faded to shiny white crescents.

A year after my mother died, a suspicious spot showed up on my mammogram. The doctor wanted a biopsy, but my insurance required a second opinion. The second doctor squinted at the film: "Yeah, it's a little strange. But let's talk odds. You drive the Nimitz Freeway to work, don't you? Well, the odds of your crashing on that freeway are a heck of a lot higher than the odds of this turning out to be cancer."

I got a third opinion and had the surgery. The lump was benign.

But there's another story, the story of my mother's internist. A good doctor, a kind man. A man who examined the lump she was worried about and sent her away several times with reassurances and no mammogram even though it had been five years since she'd had one. But that was 1986 when physicians were just beginning to be educated about breast cancer and the importance of regular mammograms.

I learned that the extra few months that passed before the mammogram was ordered almost certainly would not have altered my mother's fate. And yet. For several years after she died, I was haunted by the phrase, "what if," which joined up with my "what ifs" when she made the decision not to try more chemo and instead go home to die. Thinking of the years lost to my mother when she was so depressed and the years lost to her when she died too young, I was filled with a grief that colored my days and nights.

I'd written a few poems after my mother's death. Then more and more. I wrote on scraps of paper. The back of bills, half-written sheets from students' discarded journals. I took to carrying my Sierra Club desk calendar in my car and writing engagements in tiny print so that when the week was over I could use the leftover space for lines of poetry, lines usually composed in the traffic jam during my morning commute.

For many months my mother was at the core of each poem I wrote—poems about the last nightgown she gave me, torn and stained now but still the most precious piece of clothing I own; about the woman sorting cherries in the grocery store who looked so much like my mother I had to restrain myself from touching her; about Mother's laughing promise to haunt me so I'd know there are indeed ghosts with a sense of humor.

I tried to keep my mother's memory alive in another way, by planting an azalea on the anniversary of her death each year. The first two years, I chose beautiful red ones, tended them carefully, thrilled at the slow unbuttoning of each bud. But I am not a gardener. The responsibility of creating something beautiful outdoors and then making sure it doesn't die seems awesome to me. I have my family, my writing, my teaching. It is all I can do to nurture these parts of my life. And so my azaleas were gradually neglected, became leggy and brown. One year I forgot to plant one at all. I wept, fearing I was losing the memory of my mother.

Several years later in an M.F.A. program, I was asked to think about the direction in which my writing was going and to list the words appearing most often in my poems. I observed that my mother had disappeared as the subject for my poems, that my writing was no longer grounded in such personal loss. Yet when I looked, there they were in my poems, littered everywhere. Flowers and bones. Sweet peas, delphiniums, lilies, begonias. Phrases like "bone-flicker," "dry contour of bone," "blossom-clump on saguaro's bony arm." Lines like, "How bones glisten like stones. Little still things."

At around the same time, I discovered my mother's journals and notebooks. It was like a blessing, washing over me with a force so strong that brooding was replaced with curiosity. Instead of being consumed with her death, I learned about her life. I stepped back in time, from her exquisite art journals to her fascinating travel logs, her quirky lists and quotations, the humorous phrases she'd recorded from her children, the heartbreaking maroon notebooks. Back to a napkin from the Mermaid Cocktail Lounge where she and my father had a drink on their honeymoon. Back to sorority pledging instructions and a dance card for the Lolly Pop Charity Ball. Back to high school papers with titles like "Who am I?"

And back to the yellow pages of her high school newspaper column, *Campus Classroom Chatter,* when the world appeared fresh and exciting to her. Above the column is her picture—curled auburn hair, peter pan collar and bow, amused eyes. I read and I see that what she wrote so many years ago embodies the core of who she was when she died, in all her splendid hope and humor and intensity and love for the people and things around her:

As your campus classroom scribbler started her weekly article, with much wrinkling of brow and chewing of pencil, she suddenly sat up straight and whistled. Jeepers! This is the last time there'll be a column written by these ten busy fingers. This is it; it's graduation time! What a wonderful feeling to be going out into the world! It's been swell knowing you.

Sandra Spanier

"No communion with despair": Kay Boyle on Cancer

> Just before the deputy's key rapped sharply on the glass, Malone exhorted the President to comprehend the inevitable impatience and righteous indignation of the women of America who had, for over half a century, demonstrated peacefully for a political right. He was urging him to take action on the suffrage amendment when the deputy called out from the hall, "Lights on!" I got up carefully, carefully, from the cot, soft-footed as a cat in my outsized sneakers, so as not to awaken the girl. And Malone, too, got to his feet and said quietly: "I left the executive offices, and never saw him again." After I had turned on the switch, and taken my towel and soap from the drawer of my night table, I went to the lock-up shower, where plywood nailed across the window took the place of sawed-through bars and broken glass. It was then, as I soaped myself up and down and back and forth under the strong, warm needles of water, that I felt the lump for the first time. It was very small. It was really nothing. When I dried myself, it was still there. By six-thirty in the morning, when the cart creaked up the hall with breakfast for one and all, it had not gone away.
>
> —Kay Boyle, "Report from Lock-Up"

IN APRIL 1968 KAY BOYLE WAS IN JAIL FOR DEMON-strating against the war in Vietnam, serving a portion of her thirty-day sentence over Easter so as not to disrupt her creative writing classes at San Francisco State, when she discovered the lump in her breast. She was released from prison early on the intervention of her lawyer and on April 23 underwent a radical mastectomy. She was to live another twenty-four years until her death in 1992 at the age of ninety. Much of Kay Boyle's fiction was deeply autobiographical, from her earliest novels, drawn from her experiences in France in the 1920s among the expatriate avant-garde, to her last, *The Underground Woman* (1975), in which a writer who teaches for a living at a Bay Area college is arrested and imprisoned in a group of antiwar protesters and finds relief from her personal struggles (she has lost her husband to lung cancer and a daughter to a cult) by immersing herself in the public one. But Kay Boyle wrote publicly of her breast cancer only once—in her essay "Report from Lock-Up," which appeared along with essays by Erica Jong, Thomas Sanchez, and Henry Miller in a book called *Four Visions of America* (Capra Press, 1977). Nine years to the day after her surgery, she wrote to her publisher on April 23, 1977, that she had received her check and copies of the book. She added: "Tomorrow I go to the hospital for a cancer operation. This is the second time around, and was quite unexpected. I still have not had a moment to read the other essays in the book, but hope to do so while recuperating."

Exactly two months after her first mastectomy, on June 23, 1968, the *San Francisco Sunday Examiner and Chronicle* featured an article entitled "Kay Boyle: Genius at Large." The occasion was the publication by Doubleday of *Being Geniuses Together,* described as "a binocular view of Paris in the '20s"—a rare dual autobiography compiled and edited by Kay Boyle in which her own chapters alternate in dialogue with the resurrected memoirs of her late friend Robert McAlmon, once-influential expatriate writer and publisher, who had died nearly forgotten in Arizona in 1956. "Miss Boyle, vibrant in appearance despite recent major surgery, wore a black cotton suit that plainly said Paris, and heavy silver bracelets. Her dark auburn hair was brushed softly back from her slender, patrician face and there was an eagerness in her bright blue eyes. 'I'm glad school is out. I taught five courses and it was rugged. My jail terms were served during Christmas and Easter vacations and each week end.'" It sounds too easy in the newspaper. But it may not be fair to blame the reporter for glossing over the trauma of Kay Boyle's breast cancer. It was characteristic of Boyle to assume an undaunted air in the face of pain or illness.

Twenty years later, in the spring of 1988, the night before she was to be interviewed at her home in Oakland for the NBC *Today* show (soon after the publication of her *Life Being the Best and Other Stories*), Kay Boyle suffered an angina attack that landed her in cardiac intensive care. She insisted that the correspondent and producer come see her in the hospital the next morning, where she received her visitors with tubes in her nose and a pink chiffon scarf around her neck, wearing her trademark white earrings. She was disappointed that they were unwilling to tape an interview on the spot. "Oh dear, this was to have been my moment of triumph," she sighed self-mockingly. The interview was rescheduled and the seven-minute piece (long for morning television) broadcast on July 27, 1988.

"Report from Lock-Up" is a long meditation on the solitary confinement of the individual, in which Kay Boyle weaves together the account of her own imprisonment with other prison narratives, evoking figures as varied as anarchist Alexander Berkman, the Birdman of Alcatraz, and Alice Paul, who was jailed and force-fed in the nation's capital in the struggle for women's suffrage. Her discovery of the lump in her breast in the prison shower four-fifths of the way through the essay interrupts an imagined conversation between Woodrow Wilson and Dudley Field Malone, who went to the White House to resign his administrative post, unwilling to serve any longer in a government that denied the vote to women. The essay ends with Kay Boyle in the back seat of a police car on the way to the county hospital to be examined—the essay itself does not even reveal the diagnosis. She embeds her account of cancer in her prison narrative and in the larger context of women's history—interested not so much in exploring her personal experience with illness as in examining the health of the body politic.

Even in her private correspondence, Kay Boyle rarely devotes more than a few sentences to the subject of her health amid other matters, as in her letter of April 13, 1968, to Howard Nemerov:

Dear Howard—

I am so happy about the Guggenheim! It is never too late to get them, and then there is always a renewal coming up.

I emerged from prison four days ago (finishing up my second term), heaved a sigh of enormous relief, and then discovered I have cancer, damn it. I'm to be operated on April 23rd and I'll write you as soon after that as I can.

It was lovely of you to try to telephone me, but I'm so far from the phone (at the top of the house) that I never hear it. I have put my number at top of this letter, but I teach three nights a week so if you do call make it person-to-person.

Much love to all of you,

Kay

Characteristically, she keeps the focus on her correspondent, her tone matter-of-fact. Even when writing to tell a friend she has cancer (and she is angry about it), she begins with congratulations and ends with thoughts of his phone bill.

It would be a mistake to read this reticence as repression or denial. Rather, it seems a deliberate attempt to exert whatever control she can—coping with cancer by trying to contain it, cutting off the nourishment of attention and resisting its further encroachment into her life. Clearly, she suffered profound pain in mind and body, which she frankly expressed to friends. But her mode was to acknowledge the facts and move on. In her letters as well as in the single published essay that mentions her cancer, she nearly always discussed her illness in the context of other subjects, deflecting attention away from herself toward some practical matter, work to be done, a concern of her correspondent, or events in the tumultuous world at large.

On April 11, 1968, she wrote to her old friend Canadian writer John Glassco (who, having been born in 1909, was the "baby" of the group of expatriates she had known in the twenties and would always be "Buffy" to her): "Just yesterday, after my return home, I discovered (following examination at hospital) that I have cancer. I am to be operated on April 23rd. This was so unexpected that I'm a bit stunned, and am working like mad to get everything in order. I shall be teaching next week, and then enter hospital on April 22nd....I do hope things are going better in your life, dearest Buffy," she concludes, "and I shall be looking for word from you." (The two had been corresponding about the painful experience of his wife's struggle with schizophrenia). She also wrote that day to her agent, Armitage Watkins: "Dear Mike, It's such an unexpected business—I am to be operated for cancer on April 23rd. It infuriates me—I was released from prison on my lawyer's intervention about treatment I received there. I shall write of it one day. I'll have someone write to you as soon as operation is over. In the meantime, will you be an angel and order me from Random House I. F. Stone's *In A Time of Torment?*" In a third letter of April 11, 1968, addressed "To my Family and Executors," she takes care of another bit of business: "It is my wish to be buried in the Golden Gate National Cemetery at San Bruno, in the same grave with my late husband, Joseph M. Franckenstein. In the event that my son Ian S. Franckenstein is out of the country and cannot be present at the time of my burial, I would like Professor Herbert Wilner of San Francisco State College to read (in place of a religious service) the poetry I shall leave with him." Attached is a typewritten translation of Bertolt Brecht's poem "To Those Born Later." It begins: "What times are these when/It is almost a crime to talk of trees/For that means silence about so many evil deeds?"

In Kay Boyle's correspondence with Janet Flanner— *The New Yorker*'s "Genêt," who had testified on Kay Boyle's behalf during a McCarthy era loyalty-security trial in 1952—and Solita Solano, then living near each other in France, we can see both the sustenance Kay Boyle was able to draw from longstanding friendships and her concern for the world at large, where in the spring of 1968 students were rioting in the streets of Paris, Martin Luther King, Jr. and Robert F. Kennedy would be assassinated, and the war in Vietnam raged on. "Your letter has just this moment come—I was about to write you, sweet, good, loyal friend," Kay Boyle wrote to

Solita Solano on April 15. "Yes, Martin's death was a blow to the heart to us all." She was enclosing a photograph taken on the steps of the induction center in Oakland "a few moments before the police came in, in their flying wedge" and arrested her for civil disobedience. ("We had been sitting about six hours, and I look a bit pained. My legs were terribly stiff," she notes parenthetically). "I am glad dear Janet is better," she continues. "How I wish I could see each of you, and all of you! I have a bit of annoying news. I discovered, after my release from jail last week, that I have cancer of the breast. I am to be operated next Tuesday, April 23rd—my colleagues at San Francisco State are trying to arrange it (through appeal) that I get my salary through June even though I won't be able to go back to my job until next September."

Janet Flanner wrote from Paris on April 18 to express "our love and anger that an illness falls on you, who should be spared all physical payments except those that are voluntary, such as going to jail for all of us, or going to riots for all of us": "What a terrible two years these last ones have been with such wicked news as the assassination of Dr. King and before that month after month, year after year, of that wicked disgusting Vietnam war—How can we Americans prove to be so unreliable, so different in acts than what we talk of and claim we think and believe. This has been two years of bitter disappointment for all of us who are alike—" "Illness is also a little more costly than health," Flanner continued, and noted that she was enclosing a check that she hoped would be useful. "You are a wonderful fighting believing woman—Don't forget you are *one* of a species, without you it will become extinct!! For there is no one like you—Bless you Kay darling—If you need anything *let me know.*"

Kay Boyle responded on April 20, 1968:

dearest Janet—

In spite of the moving tenderness of your letter, my first instinct was to return the generous cheque. That I am not doing so is because the monthly payments to my beloved little mother-in-law in Austria are sometimes difficult to manage, so I have sent this great gift of yours to the Connecticut bank which sends her a draft every month. This makes my mind easier as I go to the hospital on Monday, as now she will be taken care of through May.

Your words are such welcome ones. It is not a matter of being anything exceptional or being braver than anyone else, it is simply a matter of doing what one has to do. It would be more difficult for me not to go to jail than to go. The forty days there (counting both prison terms) have been an experience I would exchange for nothing on earth—And perhaps this operation is indeed a blessing, for during the weeks of recuperation I shall have time to write—and there is so much I want to write of the jail experience, which is, in a sense, the life experience. Jimmy Baldwin flew in from Hollywood last night, where he is doing the Malcolm X script, and we talked until 2:30 this morning of all these things. It was good to have him here, and to have his most cherished ring to wear when I got to the hospital. It is good to know how much love there is—in you, in him, in all those who are like us—

Thank you, darling Janet, and know how deeply the gift is appreciated. I'll write you and Solita next week.

Ever, with devotion, and love—Kay

On April 29, 1968, Kay Boyle wrote to Solita Solano from the hospital: "This is the first day I have been able to write. The operation six days ago has seemed to have removed one quarter of my anatomy, but I'm sure it's not as bad as that. I'm still filled with tubes and contraptions which will be taken out in a few days. In the weeks ahead I will have xray treatments regularly, and I'm sure all will be well. It has been difficult, and is still extremely painful, but care is very good here and friends are wonderful—" Friends *were* wonderful. Nine years later to the day, on April 29, 1977, again in the hospital following her second mastectomy, Kay Boyle received a telegram: "THE RING IS ON YOUR FINGER COMING YOUR WAY IN TWO WEEKS ALL MY LOVE JIMMY BALDWIN."

The week of her surgery in 1968, her second husband, writer and artist Laurence Vail, father of three of her six children and of her two stepchildren (from his previous marriage to Peggy Guggenheim), died of cancer in Paris at the age of seventy-seven. "Strangely—inexplicably—I had no emotion whatever when I received the cable about Laurence's death," she wrote to Solita Solano on May 13. "Life will now be easier financially for the girls, and this rejoices me. I am feeling stronger and am religiously doing the exercises which will restore use of my arm. Tomorrow (if possible) I'll send you a copy of *Being Geniuses Together,* which will be out in June."

But if she was strangely unaffected by Vail's death, she was deeply concerned about her two youngest children, then in their twenties. That spring Ian and Faith (nicknamed "Boo" and "Mousie") were living in a Boston commune known as "the Hill" and led by Mel Lyman, author of a book entitled *Autobiography of a World Savior* and later the subject of a two-part exposé in *Rolling Stone* (David Felton, "The Lyman Family's Holy Siege of America," December 23, 1971, and January 6, 1972), which reported, among other things, that a photograph of mass murderer Charles Manson hung on the wall of the children's nursery, flowers under it changed daily. Faith had written that Kay's love for her children must also embrace Mel, and she reported that the mother of another commune member had suffered a heart attack because she was sitting in the Midwest hating the commune and its leader. But Kay Boyle flatly rejected the notion of illness as metaphor. In a letter to her son of June 5, 1968, she wrote:

> I'm sorry you and Mousie feel this cancer business is the result of some kind of wrong thinking, or lack of love, on my part. Apparently, it is (cancer of the breast) extremely likely to go from mother to daughter, and I only hope that none of my daughters will have to suffer the great pain of such an operation. I do not sit and brood over things which disturb me, as I think you know. I am, actually, much more concerned over peace in Vietnam, and over race relations, than over any personal problems. The pain of this operation—a pain which still continues, but which is marvelously relieved by strong pills—was bearable because I never ceased being aware of the pain of children being burned by napalm in Vietnam. My unhappiness over the situation on the hill is because I feel deeply about young people completely isolating themselves, alienating themselves, from their

own contemporary culture. I feel this is a great tragedy for those involved in such a withdrawal. I feel deeply about the senseless waste of energy and gifts of those who dismiss them, or belittle them [these gifts] for a group movement, and for those who impair their own identities in accepting a group identity. I do not hate any individual on the hill. I just deplore that all Mousie's great artistic gifts are being submerged, and that you are willing to submerge yours, through the acceptance of an ideology which does not for a moment reject the benefits of the materialistic world (such as money and publicity), but which appears to make a show of doing so. You know, I think, that there would be no possibility of my ceasing to love you and Mouse, as you write. But I do want all the great potentialities of you both to expand and strengthen and not to be subordinated to an individual or a group interpretation of good and evil, or success and failure. In other words, I want you both to be strong enough to find your ways of life on your own.

As I write this I am listening to the radio broadcast of what are probably Kennedy's final hours. What violence our country generates!

Robert F. Kennedy died the next day from an assassin's bullet.

While Kay Boyle usually maintained a resolutely sanguine attitude, especially in letters to her children, she was not immune from discouragement. On June 1, she wrote to Caresse Crosby, another old friend from Paris days, who with her husband Harry had founded the Black Sun Press and published Kay Boyle's first book in 1929: "The recuperation is a very slow business, and still very painful. I cannot bear being so crippled and hideous. But they tell me it is quite normal to feel this way for several months." On June 2, she wrote to Nelson Algren (whom she often called "Falcon," and whose affectionate nickname for her was "Tiger"): "I've had a bad operation, and I'm furious with life. It has relieved me of about a quarter of my anatomy, and it shows, and I am hideous, and I am going to become a recluse. It also hurts and I have to take strong pills all the time. It happened five weeks ago." She closes her letter, "Love, dear fine angry friend, Kay" and below her signature adds: "Tiger, tiger, but not shining bright." On June 26 she wrote to Solita Solano: "I am not feeling well, my dearest Solita *amie*. I have a depressing inflammation of the lymph glands in arm, and it hurts endlessly, like the mumps, and I am now told I must not typewrite (which is my life), and I waste hours soaking in hot epsom salt baths, and live on pain-killing pills—and there are moments when I feel, the hell with it all. But there is too much to be done to think of that consistently. I send you and Janet and Lib much love. I am depressed. I think of you all with tenderness."

Janet Flanner wrote again on July 1, 1968, to lend moral support: "It is *not* justice that you should be ill and in pain, you who have sought with such energy to remove pain from the lives of others in the terms of one's living and working—I am heartbroken to think of you in hospital—You can at least be sure of one thing: that you *have worked* for others' betterment, you *have been* a spirit of unselfishness and hope—of your own life you made a creation composed of the lives of others whom you did not even know personally, the thousands whose numbers represented a cause—I suppose you are a kind of saint, darling Kay....I am devoted to you by long old ties of admiration and love." Kay Boyle responded on July 10: "Thank you, beloved noble friend, for the moving statement. I carry it with me everywhere. I am looking forward so eagerly to seeing you at Christmas in Paris. (Please do not make other plans and fly elsewhere!!!) You are one of the beacons of articulated meaning and I treasure you more than you can ever know." "The pain is lessening, the arm moves more readily, and I am girding up my loins to cover the Huey P. Newton trial in Oakland," she reported. "It promises to be one of the most important trials of our period, for the whole issue of police perfidy and the meaning of black power will be deeply explored." She signs the letter with "much love" and "my gratitude for all you have testified to in the past and in the present moment."

Almost instinctively, Kay Boyle seemed to seek refuge in those requisites of mental health: love and work. Her letter of June 13 to another old friend, Bessie Breuer, who also had had breast cancer, exemplifies her ability not only to cope with grueling external demands but to tap them for strength: "While serving a second prison term at Easter I discovered a lump in my left breast. It turned out to be cancer, indeed, and at the end of April what seems to be, and feels like, my entire left side was removed. It is a long business getting back to normal (as you know well) but the use of my left arm is returning. I was able to see most of my students here at home, participate as judge in some oral examinations, and read all term papers, as well as hand in my grades for the five courses I teach. Having to do this certainly hastened my recovery." Six months after her surgery for breast cancer Kay Boyle was back in print when her "Notes on the Jury Selection in the Huey P. Newton Trial" appeared in the October 1968 issue of *The Progressive.*

In the spring of 1977, Kay Boyle had no more time for cancer than she had nine years earlier. She had taken a leave without pay from her teaching duties in order to meet the deadline for a book under contract, she was to be in New York City in February and again in April as a judge for the National Book Award, on April 13 she would deliver an address and receive an honorary degree at Skidmore College, and in May and June she was scheduled to travel to Ireland to conduct final interviews for a book on Irish women.

She is even more terse in her letters on the subject of her cancer the second time around, again seemingly determined to focus her attention on others and on her work. To her old friends Lily and George Popper she wrote on April 2, 1977: "This is to confirm our dinner date for April 10th. It is also to give you a depressing bit of news which I learned after writing to you last week. I shall have to have a cancer operation on my return from New York. I write you this rather than tell it to you when we meet, and thus the bad news will be behind us and we can talk of more pleasant things: your coming trip to Europe, etc., etc." To her friend and colleague Herb Wilner (to whom she had sent a copy of her burial instructions in 1968), she wrote on April 3:

"Couldn't the waking-up schedule through the night be something else entirely? Remember that the Sur-realistes *always* woke at two a.m. and 4 a.m. because those were the hours of highest creative potential—not to mention 6 a.m. Breton, Tzara, Jolas, and the others always had notebooks by their beds in order to write at precisely those times. Maybe it's your creative urge telling you something. I wrote three poems at 2 a.m. one day last week—Love, Kay." To Shawn Wong, a young writer and her former student at San Francisco State, she wrote on April 9, 1977: "I'm leaving tomorrow for New York (trip paid by the National Book Award) and when I get back I unfortunately have to have another cancer operation. That will take place on the 22nd. I've been thinking a lot about your novel. Have you a more recent version than the mss. I have? I thought when I get out of the hospital I could show your most up-to-date version to Capra Press and suggest I write an introduction to it."

The aftermath of her second mastectomy was particularly difficult. She was unable to swallow following the surgery, her throat damaged by the plastic tube inserted to administer anesthesia. (She was horrified and outraged at one doctor's offhanded remark that during a lengthy operation an assistant surgeon will sometimes "lean on" a patient, and she contemplated a lawsuit). But the pain was more than physical. On May 10 she wrote to Shawn Wong: "I have had a very bad time since the operation (there were complications) and am just home again, trying to get back on solid foods and gain back twenty pounds. But I did not have as bad a time as my beloved Herb Wilner, who died last Friday night after open heart surgery at Stanford. I cannot bear the senseless loss of this great man." But her determination to go on is irrepressible. The next paragraph begins: "Shawn, I feel your novel needs more work before being submitted to a publisher. I have (before the operation) gone over the opening pages and marked suggestions. I feel this book is terribly, terribly important as your statement about your life and that you should recognize that importance to your writing career. I have many constructive suggestions to make, but I fear I cannot read more of the mss. before I leave for France and Ireland on June 13th. Is there any possibility of your coming up here, at which time we could talk?" Kay Boyle made her trip as planned (though she never completed the book on Irish women). And she was proud when in 1979 Ishmael Reed's Berkeley press, Reed and Cannon Company, published Shawn Wong's first novel, *Homebase* (then the only Chinese American novel in print in the U.S.)—dedicated to Frank Chin and Kay Boyle. In the late 1970s she had hung a broadside on her door featuring the words of her friend Samuel Beckett that seemed to have served as her mantra: "I can't go on, I'll go on."

In 1991, her eighty-ninth year, three books by Kay Boyle saw publication, including her *Collected Poems,* dedicated to Shawn Wong. It includes "A Poem for Samuel Beckett," with which she opened her 1985 collection *This Is Not a Letter and Other Poems.* (She found it "terrifying" that a man as young as "Sam," her friend since 1929 and four years younger than she, should be so obsessed with death.) It begins, "I'll not discuss death with you by any name, however gently, soberly, you ask," and declares: "No past tense permitted either here or there." Her "Advice to the Old (Including Myself)," which appears for the first time in her final volume, if read broadly, seems to articulate her lifelong credo for dealing with illness and adversity:

> Do not speak of yourself (for God's sake) even when asked.
> Do not dwell on other times as different from the time
> Whose air we breathe; or recall books with broken spines
> Whose titles died with the old dreams. Do not resort to
> An alphabet of gnarled pain, but speak of the lark's wing
> Unbroken, still fluent as the tongue. Call out the names of stars
> Until their metal clangs in the enormous dark. Yodel your way
> Through fields where the dew weeps, but not you, not you.
> Have no communion with despair; and at the end,
> Take the old fury in your empty arms, sever its veins,
> And bear it fiercely, fiercely to the wild beast's lair.

Acknowledgments

I am grateful to Ian Franckenstein, Kay Boyle's son and literary executor, for permission to quote from her letters and for his generous ongoing support of my work. I am also grateful to Shawn Wong, Andrew Popper, and the following archives for access to and permission to quote from their collections of Kay Boyle's correspondence:

The Kay Boyle Papers and The Black Sun Press Archive, Special Collections/Morris Library, Southern Illinois University at Carbondale (KB to Bessie Breuer, Caresse Crosby, Ian Franckenstein, Armitage Watkins; Janet Flanner to KB)

Howard Nemerov Papers, Special Collections, Washington University Libraries

Janet Flanner/Solita Solano Papers, Manuscripts Division, Library of Congress (KB to Janet Flanner, Solita Solano)

John Glassco Fonds, National Archives of Canada, Manuscript Group 30 D 163, Volume 12, file 16, Kay Boyle to John Glassco, April 11, 1968

Herbert Wilner Papers, Rare Book and Manuscript Library, Columbia University/

Nelson Algren Collection, Division of Rare Books and Manuscripts, The Ohio State University Libraries.

Lucille Clifton

Poems

1994

i was leaving my fifty-eighth year
when a thumb of ice
stamped itself hard near my heart

you have your own story
you know about the fear the tears
the scar of disbelief

you know that the saddest lies
are the ones we tell ourselves
you know how dangerous it is

to be born with breasts
you know how dangerous it is
to wear dark skin

i was leaving my fifty-eighth year
when i woke into the winter
of a cold and mortal body

thin icicles hanging off
the one mad nipple weeping

have we not been good children
did we not inherit the earth

but you must know all about this
from your own shivering life

amazons

when the rookery of women
warriors all
each cupping one hand around
her remaining breast

daughters of dahomey
their name fierce on the planet

when they came to ask
who knows what you might have
to sacrifice   poet   amazon
there is no choice

then when they each
with one nipple lifted
beckoned to me
five generations removed

i rose
and ran to the telephone
to hear
    cancer   early detection   no
    mastectomy   not yet

there was nothing to say
my sisters swooped in a circle dance
audre was with them and i
had already written this poem

lumpectomy eve

all night i dream of lips
that nursed and nursed
and the lonely nipple

lost in loss and the need
to feed that turns at last
on itself   that will kill

its body for its hunger's sake
all night i hear the whispering
the soft

love calls you to this knife
for love   for love

all night it is the one breast
comforting the other

consulting the book of changes: radiation

each morning you will cup
your breast in your hand
    then cover it and ride
    into the federal city.

    if there are no cherry blossoms
    can there be a cherry tree?

you will arrive at the house
of lighting. even the children there
will glow in the arms of their kin.

    where is the light in one leaf
    falling?

you will wait to hear your name,
wish you were a child with kin,
wish some of the men you loved
had loved you.

    what is the splendor of one breast
    on one woman?

you will rise to the machine.
if someone should touch you now
his hand would flower.

after, you will stop to feed yourself.
you have always had to feed yourself.

    will i begin to cry?

if you do, you will cry forever.

scar

we will learn
to live together.

i will call you
ribbon of hunger
and desire
empty pocket flap
edge of before and after.

and you
what will you call me?

woman i ride
who cannot throw me
and i will not fall off.

Alicia Ostriker

❧

Scenes from a Mastectomy

*Vision: my breast as the Tabernacle. Open. My lungs like the
scrolls of the Torah. But a Torah without end whose scrolls are
imprinted and unfurled throughout time . . .*
—*Hélène Cixous,* Coming to Writing and Other Essays

The greatest kind of courage. The courage to be afraid.
—*Ibid.*

NOBODY WILL BELIEVE ME IF I SAY THIS. WHENEVER
I think of my mastectomy, I find myself smiling. As if it were a
comedy. Is it simply because I survived, and six years later I am still
glad to taste the preciousness of life? Is it that I feel like the hero of
my own drama, taking my bows?

Is it that I wrote a sequence of poems about my mastectomy,
and they turned out to be such good poems that I am grateful to
the cancer?

Is it that I was surprised by the love I received, the love I experienced, the resilience I found I possessed, the capacity for healing?
Is it that we rise, in crisis, like a wood chip lifted by a wave? Is it
that whatever doesn't kill you, as the saying goes, makes you
stronger?

Or do I smile in order not to collapse in guilty grief at the
thought of the dead?

I.

The night before we were to drive to New York for my mastectomy, we made love. To be precise: Jerry freaked out and took
himself to bed around 8 P.M., I followed, and we made love. Then

I got up, sat on the floor of my daughter Eve's empty room, stripped to the waist before her full-length mirror, and drew myself. Myself with my two complete breasts. To honor and remember. It was Jerry's suggestion to draw myself, and I had put it off and put it off. At the last minute I did it. Pen and ink. Full face. To the waist. To honor the breast on the eve of its sacrifice. Good strong drawing.

It was the second time he fell apart. The first time was the November day after I had the first mammogram, with its "suspicious" microcalcifications. The technicians showed me. I had to squint to see them, like dust spots. Dust thou art. My instantaneous internal response was that if I had to die, okay. I've lived a good life, had three beautiful children, written some good work. When I told Jerry, he said he was sure there was no real problem. Then the next day, playing squash, he slammed himself into a wall, came home white as Kleenex, wincing with pain whenever he had to move. The day after that we had him x-rayed; he'd cracked a rib. Funny ha-ha? Funny peculiar?

After that we were a team. I panicked, he reassured. I kept extremely busy. He did too. Through the radiologist's report that confirmed my need for a biopsy. Through waiting three weeks before meeting the surgeon, Alison Estabrook—she too is very busy—and another week before I can get the biopsy. I have talks and poetry readings to give at Notre Dame, Penn State, Robin's Books in Philadelphia. That last one is with my mother. I am racking up points for when I die of breast cancer and arrive at the heavenly gates. So, they'll say, checking my name off in the Big Book, what have you got to tell us? I'll be able to announce that I was a good daughter and did poetry readings with my mom. All this is a little stressful. I tell nobody. I have lower back pain for a week. At the Jewish Book Fair, I hear, again, of the illness of Susan Schnur, whom I love. Thanksgiving. Everyone is mellow, well-behaved, no arguments about politics or religion this time. And I tell nobody. But I don't want to die, I want to live, damn it.

*

Appointment with Alison Estabrook at Columbia Presbyterian Hospital. This is the same waiting room in which I wrote the poem "In the Waiting Room" ten years ago. I feel less sheer animal dread than I did then, how interesting. Is it that I have grown older and more phlegmatic? The flame of my spirit reduced to a few restless coals nearly smothered by ashes? Is it the intervention of the deaths of friends? Is it that I have accomplished enough, in this decade, in my writing, so that I feel I've done what I was put on earth to do, and could contentedly shuffle off this mortal coil, quitting while I'm ahead? You gotta know when to hold 'em, know when to fold 'em. Is it that my manuscript in progress, *The Nakedness of the Fathers,* is almost finished? (If I die, however, it will look like punishment for blasphemy, even though this is the most sacred work I have ever done.) Or is it that Jerry and I are harmonious?

Alison Estabrook is of middle height, rather fair, freckled, boyish, looks like early-to-mid-forties. White lab coat over wool dress. She speaks rapidly and technically but explains things when I ask. Sends my mammograms to her radiologist. Does a physical, finds no lumps or bumps. Radiologist (around the corner) reconfirms my need for a biopsy. I ask what the range of possibilities is. She says what the film shows is either a secretion the breast itself produces, or a ductal carcinoma in situ. A what? She explains. I ask what the statistics are. One in four you have cancer, she says plainly.

I head downtown to meet my friends Tess and Giannina, I tell them, we get drunk and see Kurasawa's *Dreams.* I don't want to die, damn it, I want to live.

Jerry and I agree to be completely open with each other. No taboos. No jokes barred. He says he will be perfectly happy if I have only one breast, as long as he still has one to hold onto. I try not to be paralyzed with dread. I tell nobody. I keep my secret fear like a bone wrapped in a handkerchief to take out and chew on when I am alone. I am perfectly normal, busy, normal, busy. Only some days, late in the afternoons, I implode, dive into bed in fetal position, become a motionless speck in a large white empty chamber whose walls, floor, and ceiling are rounded off like the inside of a freezer. A week later we drive to the city at dawn for my biopsy.

The Atchley Pavilion is entered through a vast, surreally empty lobby of polished marble, a temple of modern medicine in which the human body feels absurdly small and sticky. First stop is Radiology. I settle Jerry in the corridor and perform the ritual of undressing yet again in a tiny mammography room, where the microcalcification area has to be located with a needle and its location confirmed by a mammogram. The technician jabs the needle into the top center of my breast. I did not know this would happen; somehow I thought they would sneak it in under the breast's droop. When I emerge, Jerry is sitting outside, reading the paper, paralyzed. They wheel me off in a wheelchair to Surgery. We are right on schedule, 9:30 A.M. The Irish anesthesiologist chats me up. I'm getting a local, with a wee shot of somethin' darlin' in the I.V. to carry me through the shot of novocaine, but I ask not to have a sedative. I have hated sedatives ever since an obstetrician tricked me into having one when my son was being born and then gave me a spinal I didn't want. Never have I been more angry. We were at war in Vietnam at the time, and invaded Cambodia a few days after my son's birth. The parallel between that American military invasion of a helpless people and the doctor's invasion of my helpless body haunted me for ten years, until it became the theme of "Cambodia," the opening prose-poem of *The Mother/Child Papers.* So, so, Herr God. So, Herr Lucifer. Sylvia Plath's white fury at the experts who enjoy manipulating human bodies is something I can understand. So no sedatives, please. Consciousness. Give me consciousness. I say hi to Dr. Estabrook in her green mask. I caress my soft belly under the sheet with my free hand until they strap that hand, too, to an arm rest. No soft, random, subversive self-love allowed here. And put oxygen tubes in my nostrils. Nasty. And a curtain between me and the action, so I cannot see it, only hear it (sawing and snipping) and feel it (sensation of pressure, only slight pain, less than hitting a nerve at the dentist's). I hate not seeing. I hate being made into a blank, an exclusion. An excision. I watch the ceiling, the I.V., my cardiogram, I listen to the anesthesiologist instruct his trainee. So this is what they call minor surgery.

They have a Christmas wreath and a menorah on the counter of the recovery room, and a crepe Happy Holidays strung across it. Happy? Jerry is very happy to see me again. Estabrook has already told him all was well. She asked me, How will I recognize him? I said, He's the one who looks as if he's married to me. She didn't have a problem. He is sitting as far as possible from the room's entrance, off in a corner, buried in paper, crumbs on his tie. He asks me what made the nurse ask him if he was nervous, and I crack up.

It is a beautiful brisk December day, we are back in Princeton by 2 P.M. My wound seems not to be bleeding, as the dressing stays dry; nor does it hurt much. I don't fill the codeine prescription.

But I have been stabbed in the chest. I feel stabbed.

That was Tuesday. Wednesday I am supposed to meet Evan Zimroth in the city to go to the Genesis Seminar. It's icy cold, I wait for the 4 P.M. bus on the corner, huddling. The bus drives by me without stopping, brightly lit and full of passengers, and I burst into sobs on the street. Darkness has already fallen, not a person is in sight, the trees on the corner are black silhouettes. Tears freeze on my cheeks. I am too frightened to drive, even to the train, so I go home and phone Evan and apologize to her machine. When she calls back, I tell her. She says her mother died of breast cancer. I hang up and crawl into bed. Thursday I eat the last of the five-flavor Life Saver pack we bought Tuesday. M was supposed to visit today but it didn't work out. I am obsessed with keeping my dressing dry. Friday morning the call comes from Estabrook: the biopsy is positive. Positive. Positive means I have cancer, and I realize that until this moment I have believed it could not be so. Without even knowing it, I have passed a threshold, crossed a border, become a permanent citizen of the nation of fear. It is as if a coat of ice has formed around me. What must I do now? What is the recommended treatment? It will be either a wider excision and radiation, or mastectomy, depending on how widespread the cancer is, Estabrook says. My husband and I must come to confer with her. I ask her secretary to schedule me for that conference, and for an appointment with a reconstructive surgeon, and for the surgery itself as soon as possible. I want this done. I want speed. It is imperative to have the surgery in time so that I can go back to work teaching second semester. I call Jerry at work. Oh baby, he says, poor baby. He asks me if he should come home but I say no, no, I'm all right, only I do not know if I should have one kind of surgery or the other. He says he will support me in whatever I choose. I call my best girlfriend Sheila. She will try to locate her friend Bev who had a mastectomy fifteen years ago. An old friend with whom I share poetry phones me from work, but I tell him I can't talk with other people around. He calls back from home, and I tell him. I hear the silence on the phone, then he says he will be right over. An hour later he shows up with Joni Mitchell and Bonnie Raitt tapes. We talk about my diagnosis, and his poems, and he is more than friendly, he is tender. He says how alive I look. He tells me today is the fifth anniversary of his sister's death from leukemia. Finally, such is his compassion, he raises the subject of how we made love once (twice, I correct him) years ago and have never spoken of it since. Because I'm shy, I say. He says he guesses he's shy too. And because, I say, I figured it was more important for me than for him. He says it was important for him too. A sweet talk, and it ends with kissing goodbye at the door, real kisses. His soft blond hair falls over my face.

Estabrook phones again. She recommends mastectomy, not a wider excision, because my ducts are "crawling with cancer cells."

*

I am determined to tell everyone now. Jerry agrees. Tell, don't hide. But also live my life, our lives, as normally as possible. I love this particular life I have chosen, my teaching, my writing, my husband. This is the house which I have built. Here is the earth on which I stand. Whatever my hand findeth to do, let me do it with my might. Let me not become swallowed up by cancer. I don't want to be eaten alive, I refuse. I resolve to keep extremely busy. I work on my Whitman essay, on letters of recommendation, on Christmas and Chanukah cards. I buy the new edition of *Our Bodies, Ourselves.* It is terrifying. Jerry is terrified too. Later we realize there's nothing in it about DCIS (ductal cancer in situ), which is what I have, and which is the fastest-growing area of cancer studies because the technology of mammography now enables diagnosis to occur without a lump. Over the weekend I begin the phone calls. Feels like millions of them. Filaments and ganglia of connection reveal themselves. Paths branch toward further paths. Everyone puts me in touch with someone else. Everyone is so kind, so generous, it is a gift. Each new human contact is like a warm penny pressed against the icy window of my spirit, melting a spot, turning it from cold white to blurry swimming color. For a few moments each time I can see through these circles, soft browns and blues, colors of life, then I freeze over again.

Wednesday afternoon we have conferences with Dr. Estabrook and with Dr. S, the plastic surgeon. An hour wait in Dr. S's waiting room, reading the current (DO NOT REMOVE FROM THIS OFFICE) *Newsweek,* December 10, 1990, with a photograph of President Bush gritting his teeth and making two fists, one on either side of the microphone. "This Will Not Be Another Vietnam." Translation: I am not a wimp. We are preparing to go to war in the Persian Gulf. And another cover story: "The Politics of Breast Cancer: A Fight Over Treatment and Money."

Dr. S is a nice brown-eyed Jewish boy, went to Brandeis like me. He explains the two kinds of reconstruction, saline implant (they

no longer use silicone) and self-tissue reconstruction using material taken from one's belly. This is ingenious: an oval of skin, and the
attached fatty tissue, is pulled up on the inside, then molded on
the chest with its own blood vessels still attached. It can be
sculpted like one's own breast, which an implant cannot. We discuss advantages and disadvantages, he examines me in his consulting room and at one point puts his hand reassuringly on my knee.
Who needs this? I am slightly inclined to kick him in the jaw. The
photographs of reconstructed ladies make me feel a little like
throwing up. These do not look like real breasts. They look scarred
and lumpy. Breasts made of kindergartener's Play-Doh. *My body is
speaking to me. It is throwing me images of a body with a breast on
one side and a boy's chest on the other. See? It's pleading. Not so bad?
Rather nice?* Reconstructive surgery requires several visits for an
implant, then you probably get the other breast "fixed" to match
the new one, which is adolescently round. Self-tissue means more
pain, several weeks to heal. Probably I would be unable to return
to work second semester. And more danger of infection. And your
stomach muscles are weakened forever. Who needs this? If before
this appointment I was veering toward the hey-presto magic of
one-procedure reconstruction, the idea of waking up as if nothing
had happened, I am certainly back-pedaling now. Something is
going to happen. I am going to lose a breast. In real life, in real
time. Unless I opt at the last minute for wider excision instead of
the mastectomy. And I do not want something stuck on me/in me
that will mask the reality. Suddenly I don't want everything to be
nice and normal. No, I want truth. *My body is sending me pictures.
Fish, stabbed fish, healed over, swimming in deep water. Half-boy,
half-woman.* I ask Dr. S if he will give me names of past patients.
He agrees but forgets. I think I will put reconstruction on hold.

   I had asked Dr. Estabrook for recommended reading. She hands
us four articles from 1988-89 medical journals, all on DCIS. It is
pushing 7 P.M. We huddle on a sofa in her empty waiting room.
Somewhere out in the world night is falling, cars and buses and

taxis are flowing along Broadway, the subway is rumbling through its tunnel. We sit here under fluorescent lights cocooned in a timeless space. Jerry races through the articles, he is accustomed to reading scientific literature, I plod behind. He extracts the idea that a wider excision, plus radiation plus monitoring plus a mastectomy if there is a recurrence, gives you the same 100 percent survival rate as an initial mastectomy. He keeps showing me the table with the zero deaths. My brain feels turned to snow. I ask Estabrook about this possibility, but she resists, because 1) my cancer is "extensive," and 2) radiation thickens tissue and makes it harder to spot recurrences or lumps. Jerry says what about this table with the zero deaths.

The question remains unresolved. The decision I had thought was (ha-ha) clear-cut, isn't. I am still on overdrive, my brain is still snowing.

Second opinion in the morning: Dr. O at Memorial Sloan-Kettering. It is more like a factory here than Columbia Presbyterian. A sweatshop. One whole floor is devoted to financial arrangements. You sit in a cubicle while a smiling clerk enters your vital statistics, especially those pertaining to insurance, into her computer. The process should take two minutes but takes twenty. You feel as if you are on a welfare line trying to prove your worthiness for some sort of aid you never asked for. Around Dr. O's office it is more like Bloomingdale's. Jammed with women in white plastic chairs up against a wall, women alone or with their husbands, all with cancer on their minds beneath their hairdos, between their fourteen-karat gold earrings. Dr. O flits by periodically, the master of the revels, radiating intelligence and charm.

He charms me at first, then less and less. British, slender, olive-complexioned, attractive, gracious. Speaks of his accent with slight self-mockery. Went to Oxford. Chats me up about my work, asks if I publish, says he did English for a while. Says he has a shelf of books given to him by patients. I make the crude blunder of asking innocently if he has read them; he evades, repeats, "You can't *imagine* what an array I have!" I mention who referred me to him and his eyes light up: "A marvelous woman! And her husband contributes scads of money for my research!" Alison Estabrook is "one of us; there are really very few of us in New York, actually, seven here, five there." But I am here to get a second opinion on my cancer, on whether to have mastectomy or a wider excision, not to flatter or be flattered. "What you have shouldn't be called a cancer," he says emphatically. "It's a condition." The point is that it is not a cancer until it is invasive? And it might remain dormant forever? So what, I think, this is semantic. He runs through the advantages and disadvantages of my two options. The mastectomy is 100 percent sure (everyone converges on this) but you have "disfigurement." Wider excision risks recurrence. We talk statistics awhile, the research being done in France; the bottom line is that Dr. O prefers not to make a clear recommendation. Reasonable, I suppose, but disappointing. Why have I spent my morning here? Not to mention his doubtless astonishing fee, which my insurance will only partially cover. I note also that he assumes I want reconstruction and seems a bit put out when I say I'm not sure I do. And he becomes quite cross when I say I'm in a hurry and want to be done so that I can be back teaching in January.

I go home exhausted, confused. Sheila calls me every day. My sister calls to say she is coming with her son Kyle for New Year's. She has a lump near her nipple. Tess has a lump. Fear is like snow, like a blizzard. Numbed, I push myself through it day by day, as it whips at my face, sticks to me, stings and congeals.

Friday morning, we are in the countdown and still have not decided. Two more second opinions scheduled. I am almost certain that it is the mastectomy I want. Jerry is the gambler, the poker player, the motorcyclist. He thinks if it were his body he would take a chance. My personality is risk-averse. We drive back to the city. Dr. K was Sue B's surgeon. His is an old-fashioned, non-high-tech building and office; he's an older man, probably near retirement. Jerry and I glance at each other as we introduce ourselves to him. Both of us feel comfortable with this gentleman and his slightly soft green chairs and settee. We chat a little. Amusingly, he too apparently needs to establish his credentials. He remarks that he is on the academy committee selecting papers for a forthcoming conference. He recalls that Alison Estabrook submitted one but he has not read it yet. Like Dr. O, when we move into the issue of what kind of surgery would be best for me, he wants to be noncommittal. But we don't leave, we keep asking questions. He talks to Jerry automatically and has to keep reminding himself to address me, the patient in question. Finally he says, impatiently, that he doesn't care what these researchers claim (Understood: *young* researchers). Once you have a palpable cancer your chances are fifty-fifty. He talks of a dying woman patient who is suicidal. At last he says, when pressed, "If it were my wife, I'd choose mastectomy." Good. I write a check for $200, or is it $220, for his time, I cancel the other appointment, we drive up to see Estabrook one last time with a few more questions. And that's that. I feel secure in her office. It's minimal. It has a view of Amsterdam Avenue. I feel at home here. We've made our decision.

We murmur, driving home, leaning together as we ascend the spiraling ramp toward the George Washington Bridge, of how magic this time has been for us, how intimate we have become. It is as if a door had opened between us. The door between two worlds, as the poet Rumi calls it. You must ask, Rumi says, for what you really want. The New Jersey Turnpike slides by. Jets pass overhead on their way to Newark Airport. We wonder how we can retain this magic when the crisis is over. I leave Jerry at work and drive to Quaker Bridge Mall, blazing with energy. I buy everyone's Christmas presents in a shower of adrenalin. Sweaters for Rebecca and Eve, moose slippers for Nat, a silk and wool opera scarf and a Bah Humbug shirt for Jerry, a cookbook and spices for Gabe to support his cooking habit. It's dark when I leave. Dark and cold. Stinging winter air. And I'm sweating and exhausted. I have trouble finding the car in the unreal wasteland of the mall parking lot. I fear I'll catch a cold and have to miss my surgery next Tuesday.

*

Magic? I cannot begin to describe how good a husband and friend Jerry has been to me during these days and weeks. Steadfastly available when I need him. Insisting that he knows I will be fine. Insisting that whatever decision I make is fine with him. He treats me as if I am strong, not weak, and this strengthens me. We make love almost every day now. But the main thing is that we have agreed to be completely open with each other, to say whatever comes to mind. Even "crazy" things. His first thought when I came home with the mammogram news, he says, was "Lop the damn thing off." I like that. He says he will be altogether contented as long as I have one breast to offer him. If I didn't have any, he would put the ad in the *New York Review of Books*. Short dark Jewish scientist seeks short dark Jewish poet or nursery school teacher for friendship and intimacy. Must have at least one breast. We joke about this ad a lot. It's an old family joke, inventing these personal ads. I compose variations. One morning he points out to me that the mode I am in—survival mode, he calls it—is like the way I set my goals of self-healing, and attained them, after I was raped, fifteen years ago. I am astonished that he says this. It is perfectly true, but that rape is an episode he has tried to erase from his consciousness. As for me, I tell him whatever swims into my mind. *I see myself as a fish. I see myself as Amazon, as androgyne. I remember the pillared stone bas-relief of the androgynous god Shiva, one palm facing outward, one arm flung around a buffalo neck, torso gracefully curved, a male chest on his left side and a breast on his right, carved in the living rock of the cave temple on the Island of Elephanta. The holiest place on earth I have ever been.*

We talk in bed each morning. One morning I say: We could pickle the breast and put it in a jar. He says: a Mason jar. I say: I could paint a face on it.

Another morning I say: *I want to say farewell to my breast. It's alive, it is an entity, it doesn't want to die. I want to thank it for all its kindness to me for so many years. Like a Navaho thanking the deer for surrendering its life. I want to say a prayer or have a ritual.* He turns away in bed. That would make me grieve, he says, meaning no, this is one game he does not wish to play with me. I say: *Grief is inevitable, I thought I could modify it by doing some of the grieving beforehand. I can hear my breast crying, like a baby. It blames me and calls me selfish. I am a selfish, cold-hearted killer.* He does not answer. I do not push. We are being tolerant of each other. We are making love almost every night. I am very in love with my husband. He turns over on the pillow. You could draw yourself, he says. Do a self-portrait.

The husband of a woman we know who was diagnosed with breast cancer ordered her not to tell anyone. He didn't want to be pitied by his colleagues. Nice? May he rot in hell.

Of the kids, I told Eve first. Called her the weekend after the biopsy report. My line was: With a mastectomy I get 100 percent twenty-year survival, I can't even get hit by a truck, I thought I was immortal before but now I *really* will be. She bit. You can hear when someone is stunned on the phone, and she was, but she came right back, caught the (cheerful, normal, let's joke please) tone I wanted, and reproduced it heroically. As soon as she hung up, she doubtless went bawling to Nat. Next day she called Jerry at work and he gave her the reassurance speech. Rebecca took it harder; she couldn't joke, she couldn't talk. My fault, probably—I had been trying to reach her all weekend but she was away at a wedding, I had to call her at work and was feeling panicky at the moment I reached her, had no bright strategy but blurted out my news. She would have no place to hide, in her office surrounded by co-workers. Without a door to shut on them if she wanted to. Oh my beloved girl, I am sorry. Forgive me.

Calling Gabe was hardest. A twenty-year-old boy struggling to find his identity, troubled over his coursework, in the middle of exams, tender and sensitive of spirit—how could I burden him with this information? How could I say, Oh, by the way, when you come home for break I'll be in hospital minus a breast? I delayed and delayed and finally could delay no longer. My strategy was to chat, first, of pleasant things like taping Indian music for him; hear his news; then tell. I was so frightened. But this boy was unbelievable. I made my speech, could hear his silent shock, like a windowshade pulled down, very briefly—then he rallied in a way that I could never have predicted yet was perfectly appropriate to him: he asked me questions. Of course. The windowshade flew up in an eyeblink. How long would the surgery take, what kind of anesthetic, what exactly was the diagnosis, how long would I be in hospital? He was, in other words, himself—of all our children, the one with the liveliest curiosity. And a boy no longer, but a man, a mensch. How proud I was of him. And a day later—oh, my heart—he called with a set speech. "Mom, it doesn't matter if you have two breasts, or one, or none, or three. I love you just the same and you're the best mom in the world."

It is the weekend before my mastectomy. It is important not to say hospitalization, not to say surgery, but to say mastectomy. The technical, the clear, the precise word. I fight to say it, not to be ashamed. To love myself courageously I must say mastectomy plainly. I go to Clayton's and buy hot pink pajamas for the hospital, satiny with soft flannel inside. They will be part of my fight to love myself. They will make me look sleek and gorgeous. On the phone to a dozen people, I am told a dozen stories, heroic, pathetic, infuriating. One woman's survival for years beyond what the doctors told her she would have. Another woman's experience of waking up without a breast when she thought she was merely receiving a biopsy. Stories of lumps the size of golf balls materializing overnight. Stories involving pus, blood, vomit. Stories about women organizing to demand more research into the causes of breast cancer. Women on chemo, women covering or refusing to cover their baldness. These are the invisible webs women weave together. We spin our secret filaments, filiations, out of the earshot of men. Men who would be scandalized, men who would be horrified to hear us speak as we do about our bodies. To hear us speak, cackle, whisper, and roar as we do about birth, about sex, about sickness. Men who are afraid of blood. Centuries, millennia, of women's secrets, forced into secrecy by men's dread of our bleeding. Of the phantoms we live among, perhaps the greatest, the oldest, is the colossus of the bloody goddess. Invisible to her children, she bestrides civilization. Her body empties itself and heals but is never closed, it pours forth milk and blood continuously, and we rational beings cannot bear it. We refuse her worship. We pretend she does not exist. The talk that circulates among women—the private telling—is a faint echo of a once-universal psalm of praise and fear, now indescribable.

II.

The sky is low, the clouds are mean. A few flakes of snow hang in the air. Now the horizon shifts from tar black to transparence, red juice spilling upward. Dawn breaks, icy, as we approach New York. We are driving over the bridge, contemplating once again the majestic parabola of the cables, the welter of river, the pure stony jaw of Manhattan.

The huge lobby of Columbia Presbyterian resoundingly empty. In a waiting room I give my insurance information and surrender my jewelry to a pale and harrowed Jerry, receiving in exchange a plastic bracelet with my name on it. In a locker room I denude myself, don a limp cotton hospital nightie and paper slippers to shuffle in. And wait, like a limp leaf.

Horizontal on the stretcher pushed by an orderly—why a stretcher? Why can't I walk? Or sit with dignity in a wheelchair? Why can't the anesthesiologist who has just given me the explanatory talk push me? Is maximal humiliation the intention?—I watch ceilings and corridors slide endlessly by, recalling how often I have seen others in this sad position.

Now I am one of them. An object. I have no fight at all. In the bright operating room, beneath the buzzing overhead lamps, I explain to Dr. Estabrook, as I have to everyone else, that it's my heart I'm really worried about with my family history, I hope they'll keep an eye on it. I hope they will see me as special. Ah, now they attach me to the intravenous.

Fins upon a current, lightless, swimming and supping, circling easily, downward to the silted corrugated seafloor, rocked by indifferent wavelets, held by infinite hands, imaginary orchard unfolding, capillary motion from mud upward, salt-sweet threaded to hard nubs, swollen to gold, orange lanterns against the teeming green, unfalling, uncut fruit—

—My husband at bedfoot, beautiful. Released.

A hospital is another world, and four days an aeon. Time becomes ingeniously elastic. Periodically you shuffle to and from the toilet. Meals materialize periodically, containing far too much meat. Doctors speed through as if on roller blades, nurses pop in to check vital signs like wooden figures in a cuckoo clock. Flowers, friends, family appear. My radiant children. Chocolates, balloons, fresh fruit, a packet of sugar cubes, a basket of powders, oils, and lotions, a pair of pretty earrings, love. You take as little of the codeine as possible but it's still a haze, a daze. You push the buttons to incline your bed into and out of sitting position. The phone rings and rings and you practice reaching your left arm for it. Roommates come and disappear, one night the woman in the bed next to you moans intermittently with a sound like love moans. In the next room is a young man whose ring finger was severed when he fell climbing over a railing and his ring caught. He is a musician. He needs that finger. They did microsurgery to reattach the finger, and to make blood flow from the rest of the hand into that finger they've used leeches. A leech at the tip of the finger sucks the blood on up, simple hydraulics. Channel Nine arrives and departs. You shuffle to the boy's room, your first outing, he looks about the age of your son, a thin Spanish-speaking boy with his stocky father, the two of them shining like lamps, going home today after a month here. The boy plays keyboard in a gospel band. No, he hasn't made pets of the leeches. Each time one was swollen full, it was his job to pluck it off and drop it in a bottle of alcohol.

The litter rises around you, you read three novels and write stacks of greeting cards, using Gabe's lovely computer design of a wide field, and a house, and star-shaped snowflakes, captioned PEACE. The irony leaks like a draining wound. How to write a message of hope for the new year, as we stand once again at the brim of war? The boys with toys are at the ready. *Newsweek* features photos of phallic fighter planes on the deck of USS *Midway* and a fan of pointed Hawk missiles threatening the desert sky. Some think tank ponders the possibility of Iraq using chemical weapons, in which case we would be forced to reply with a nuclear strike. Forced to reply, they actually said that. The President rattles his manly sabers. He is going to kick Saddam's ass. The *New York Times* reports: 52 percent of those polled approve the President's conduct: 57 percent want to commit troops to the Gulf; 45 percent want to commit troops only if the war is short and the casualties few. Opposition is found among many blacks. Surprise, surprise. A third of the troops on active duty in the Gulf are black. But half a dozen retired generals and admirals, and even Henry Kissinger, counsel a continued blockade rather than war. Perhaps the inevitable will not happen.

Bev brings a breast form and shows me her incision. It is necessary to look. Strangely I think of Marianne Moore's line in "In Distrust of Merits," her great World War II poem, "O/quiet form upon the dust, I cannot/look and yet I must." How she breaks the line because the world is broken and her heart is. How the poem ascends into self-accusation: "I inwardly did nothing./O Iscariotlike crime!/Beauty is everlasting/and dust is for a time." It is a poem for which many eminent critics have expressed so much contempt that you no longer see it in anthologies. Eve brings a voluptuous velvet paisley robe and an all-day sucker. Jerry brings a Dior nightie and robe. My mom brings her bewilderment. I drag Jerry into the bathroom and undo his fly, yes, I don't care if everyone in the room guesses what we are doing, yes, let them.

I cannot actually move very much. Gradually I walk. To the bathroom, to the nurse's station, finally around the whole floor. There is no sensation in my left armpit and half my left arm. Dear God, please, I hate this, do not let me be dumb numb rubber forever. Gradually, gingerly, I gather the courage to look at my wound. At first I cannot. When a doctor comes to check the dressing I avert my eyes. Then I look. Steady on. Finally I undress in the bathroom to wash. I have to hold onto the drain coming out of my side as well as look at my flat bandaged chest. Breathe deep, like a singer, like a runner, and lift the dressing. There is the long, fat, red, slimy diagonal.

Dr. Estabrook is off on vacation. I've given her a copy of *Green Age* and she looks really pleased. When I show her the cover photo of me by Jerry, she says, He was so funny. He said he had no more questions and then he had ten more. That's him, I say.

Do not hide, do not be ashamed. Think of Deena Metzger's poster, her nude arms flung above her head, the sky behind her, the snake tattoo upon the right side of her chest. What is real is reality. I will not get myself tattooed but I will not be reconstructed either. Now I am this shape, it is what I am, damn it to hell. The physical therapists visit, teach me exercises, give me a puff of lambswool to stuff in my bra. After they leave I attempt to put the lambswool in the bra cup but I cannot do it the first time. I just cannot. My hands will not obey me. I put my pajama top back on and wait a few hours, and the second time I try, I can do it.

I have been here since Tuesday. Today, Saturday, I am to go home. A crewcut doctor comes to pull my drain. Pull my plug, I think shakily. At the last minute fear drops over me again like a shroud. In a hospital, although as many Americans die each year of hospital-acquired infections as of auto accidents, one has the illusion of safety.

Jerry's secretary Irene has instructed me to languish when I get home, but I don't feel like languishing. I make breakfast for everyone the second morning I'm home, wearing the voluptuous velvet bathrobe and the hot pink pajamas beneath. I am still in overdrive. Then my wound begins to swell, and it hurts, and is a horrible wet wobble under my skin. The incision, as the scab starts peeling, grows red and infected. Jerry says I shouldn't have taken a bath. I treat it with Bacitracin and clumsy makeshift dressings. In bed I try to find comfortable positions for lying with Jerry. If I face his back I cannot rest my head on my left arm but must fold the arm under me like a chicken wing. But having my children here is so wonderful I cannot express it, everyone behaves affectionately not only to me but to each other, no fighting no biting, we make a fire each evening and sit around listening to music or playing Scrabble. Jerry is so mellow I'm almost reluctant to give him his Bah Humbug shirt at the end of our gift exchange.

I cannot sweep or vacuum. The infection heals too slowly. We have our annual New Year's Eve open house, physicists and poets, neighbors and family and students, my mom, my sister Amy flies in from California, my cousin Sylvia drives from Long Island, everyone brings dishes and old records and tapes for dancing. I want them all to see me! See how strong I am! Damn it, see how sexy I am! From Joan Wood there arrived in the mail the black-and-red silk Chinese jacket I admired on her, bearing a note: This old thing just wants to party itself to death. I wear it with black tights and high patent leather heels, damn it. I look great. I look normal! I can scarcely dance, except for my mom's obligatory folk dance session, and I don't linger in the kitchen with the rowdies. But I stick it out somehow until half past one, the party still going strong. I watch my daughter Rebecca dance. I wish she would sing too, and play her bass. The spirit in her compact body could make devils sprout wings. My prayers are for Gabe to find a girlfriend in the crowd, and for my freespirited daughter Rebecca and her ironic boyfriend Ian to snuggle well in her childhood bed.

I hate it that it hurts. I hate it that I have lost sensation in and around my armpit. I hate the disgusting scar, wet, red. A worm. A lolling stupid tongue. A scarlet letter but without a meaning. Nothing.

One of the balloons says "Get Well." One says "This balloon contains Heal-ium." They are dying slowly. Jerry promises when they are all dead my incision will be all healed. They have been floating through the house behaving like individuals. A pair monitors us in bed. One wanted to spend the night in our bathroom but I wouldn't let it. One flew from Jerry when he was chasing it and hid behind the tropical plant Martha Nell and Marilee sent. I do my exercises and hope that soon I will be able to lift my arm above my head. Oh a rainbow of passions: self-pity, self-hatred, loathing of anyone who pities me, amazed gratitude toward anyone who loves me, determination to be strong, determination to be ordinary. Damn it. I have not yet made the trip to Edith's Lingerie for my prosthesis.

The evening of Wednesday, January 16, I was in New York attending the Genesis Seminar at the Jewish Theological Seminary with Evan Zimroth. Security checked our I.D.'s at the entrance. As the meeting broke up a custodian told us that the bombs were flying. I tried to phone home without success. Walking me back to my car Evan asked me how I felt. I said that I felt like the sybil in *The Waste Land.* Evan is another poet, so she knew what I meant. We walked without speaking for another half block. The night was clear and crisp, the sky above upper Broadway seemed exalted. *I wish I had not lived to see this.* I did not plan to say that, but the words burst from my lips. After more than a decade in which my country has not been at war, except for the cowardly actions in Grenada and Panama, and of course the support of the contras in

Nicaragua and the covert CIA-sponsored overthrow of Allende. Of course there was our secret training of South American secret police, teaching techniques of interrogation, torture, and drug-running. But at least, subsequent to the Vietnam War, we have not overtly and flagrantly engaged in another large-scale imperialist action. And now our bombs will affirm our national addiction to low-priced oil, and I cannot pretend that I am glad to be an American. *I wish I had not lived to see this.* I said it again to Eve on the phone the next night. I could not prevent myself. Eve commanded me to take it back. "Say 'I take it back' ten times," she ordered, and I obeyed. Now I am memorizing W. H. Auden's "September 1, 1929," and I cannot stop crying.

Iraq bombed Israel last night. The telephone lines to our friends in Tel Aviv are jammed. Meanwhile on CNN they show again and again the shot of the same smart bomb going down the airshaft of the Defense Ministry in Baghdad. Bring on the special effects. To prevent repetition of the free media coverage of Vietnam, which helped to foreshorten that war, journalists are to be "pooled," to be accompanied at all times by military escorts, and subject to military censorship. They are not to enter the war zone. They are not to photograph any wounded or dead people. Oh, well, that should take care of everything.

As soon as I am able to touch it, I resolve to caress this flatness. My chest, my dead-feeling armpit, my arm, all that remains. I run my fingers over the area, petting it, caressing it, letting it know that I am not angry, that it is still my body, that I still love it. I tell a friend that I am doing this, caressing the place where there is no longer a breast, for which there is no name. I press my fingers gently all around the scar, I squeeze my armpit. My friend is surprised.

But if I cannot love my body, I cannot heal.

Weeks go by. The President's popularity shot from forty-some-thing percent to ninety percent in the polls as soon as he began killing people. Nobody is willing to say this simple thing. The war goes on, the images on television remain sanitized, technological, clean. It is a clean war. The term *surgical strike* is used. Our puppets recite their irrelevant lines, and the *New York Times* prints what it is ordered to print. There is virtually no coverage of the protests occuring on and around campuses. Air war turns into ground war. Yellow ribbons adorn cars and mailboxes everywhere, the whole country has turned itself into a fat satin flower. Support our boys! Could we support them by bringing them home? Nobody is willing to say what is so obviously the case, that the people of America are experiencing a communal joy over this war, and that their joy is a function of being permitted to hate a simple single enemy, Saddam Hussein, consciously, while knowing—surely knowing, just beneath the threshold of consciousness—that the war is not clean at all, not surgical, that we are in fact killing civilians, that we are killing soldiers who did not ask to be soldiers. In the end our tanks will have rolled over and buried alive, according to some estimates, as many as two hundred thousand Iraqi boys. Perhaps it was merely a hundred thousand.

The population of Iraq is just 16 million people, making it only slightly more populous than Nicaragua. So we have done what we do best: gone in with overwhelming technological and manpower superiority and defeated someone small. I must cling to accuracy in language, in this age of euphemistic rot when the War Department has become the Department of Defense and we live in a verbal drizzle of acceptable losses, collateral damage, deterrent, non-combatant, smart weapon, friendly fire, body count, strategic target, mutually assured destruction. Surgical strike.

Somewhere in the sands of the desert. A gaze blank and pitiless as the sun. The tanks rolled, blank and pitiless, leaving here and there a dead wrist, a foot in its uniform, thrust from the sand into the sunny air. But of course Yeats's poem, "The Second Coming," attempts to describe an apocalyptic transformation of history, and the Gulf War is not apocalyptic at all. It is a tiny war, a speck of a war. Like the insignificant speck of cancer in my breast a few months ago.

Between the forces arrayed against us within our own cells, and the forces of human nature acted out on the scale of human history, each of us is almost entirely helpless. Almost entirely. I have repeated "September 1, 1929" so often to myself these last few months, thinking how wrong Auden was to decide, later, that poetry makes nothing happen and to exclude that poem from his collected works. "All that I have is a voice / To undo the folded lie." Teaching my classes this semester with especial vehemence, I have attempted to offer my students the belief that although we can perhaps do little to heal either the world or ourselves, we can do *something*. Something is not the same as nothing. I teach my course in women's poetry, and my seminar, "The Bible and Feminist Imagination," in the conviction that "the laws of history," as Adrienne Rich calls them, may change very slowly and may require all the strength and ingenuity of all our lives to change them but must change in time. "If one woman told the truth about her life," Muriel Rukeyser wrote, "the world would split open." I work on my Bible book, *The Nakedness of the Fathers*, trying to locate, between and behind the compelling tales of the patriarchs and warriors, the kings and prophets, the faint traces of women's power, of goddess worship before the worship of God, almost erased from memory but still perhaps recoverable.

Once I began wearing the falsie inside my left bra cup, Jerry made a habit of hugging me, squeezing one breast or the other, and saying, "Is this the real one? I can't tell the difference." Dear Jerry. In bed he fondles the one that remains, and insists that one is just as good as two. I make it a habit to look at myself nude in the mirror until I no longer flinch. I continue to caress my own body, the flat as well as the round, the numb armpit that begins almost to know when it is being squeezed. Sheila's friend Bev calls to check on me and reminds me that a woman is really the same person after a mastectomy as before. Bev, I reply, you are so good to call. Thank you. She says the wrinkles in her face make her feel worse than the missing breast.

The biblical King David, when his infant son fell ill, fasted and wept, praying for the child's recovery. When informed after seven days that the infant had died, he rose, dressed himself in fine, fresh raiment, and ate heartily. His courtiers were scandalized, but the king explained: "While the child was alive, I fasted and wept, thinking perhaps the Lord will have pity on me and let him live. But now that he is dead, can I bring him back again? I shall go to him, but he shall not return to me." In the same way, I mourned and wept for my breast before I lost it, and when it was gone, I set my spirit to healing. And I do heal. Physically I can move around swiftly now, and my arm can do almost everything it could before. Yet as I grow stronger, I become haunted by an image of the lost breast. Where is it, where did it go? I imagine it floating down the brackish Hudson River toward the ocean, in a sort of perpetual journey, accompanied by weeds, fish, other flotsam, perhaps other portions of beings severed from their owners, their bodies that loved them, perhaps the soft forms of aborted fetuses riding the current. The jelly of a breast seems like a small child who is lost and crying for its mother. Afar off, I, its mother, can hear it cry and whimper. The sound peals backward toward me through the river waters. It is like the sound of the church bells in a poem by A. E. Housman, heard by the lover mourning his dead bride, and responding, "Oh, noisy bells, be dumb; / I hear you, I will come." So I understand that my lost breast will not return to me, but I will go to it.

Memorial Day weekend we spend in Chester, Massachusetts, at our place in the country. Gabe, who is our official sauna master, has fired up the woodstove in the sauna, and tells Jerry and me that it is almost ready. We built this sauna with our own hands, as we built this brick house up this dirt road in the middle of the Berkshires. The sauna is a decade old, tiny and fragrant. I have lately rubbed its redwood benches with lemon oil. Traditionally we sauna and plunge into the pond nude—we, our friends, our children, and our friends' children—although during their school years the children saw fit to protect their modesty with bathing suits. And so I am anxious. It will be my first time coming out, as it were. Shame and fear half choke me. Taking Gabe aside, on the path to the sauna, I remind him of a conversation months ago when I was still considering reconstruction. "I decided not to do it," I tell him. "I need to warn you that I'm unreconstructed." Once again he doesn't miss a beat. "No problem," says my boy, my young man. "You can have as many breasts as you want to, or as few." So the three of us enter the sauna, Jerry and I on one bench, Gabe on the bench opposite, laying our cotton robes aside in the dry hot shadows, and begin to sweat. Gabe throws water on the stones, steam rushes up hissing, and fills the little sauna. After a few minutes Jerry leaves, letting me and my son sit quietly, meditatively, sweating, melting, becoming at ease. I can hardly believe my luck, I sit with my legs dangling, sweat pours down my face and body but what really melts me is gratitude.

We are joined in the evening by a pack of family and friends. The weekend is raucous. When everyone leaves on Monday, I stay. It will be my first period of solitude since the surgery. The afternoon is bright, I set a blanket out on the grass, I listen to birdsong, I take my shirt off and for the first time, I touch my scar. I run my finger over its rubbery length. Slightly ridged, thickened, a flaw. A quiet worm delivered by the cosmos and permanently attached to me. The pond sparkles, the trees at the wood's edge stir slightly, I sit and let my breath slow down, I try to let my mind decelerate. No longer do I need to be tense and in control, speeding through my vigilant days and weeks as if a moment's relaxation would bring some nameless disaster. I can let go. The irises along the brim of the pond are about to lift themselves from their membranes into purple bloom. I would like to pause and remember everything. Let images float from the bottom of my mind's pond to the surface. Remember the joy and power I felt as an adolescent when my breasts finally began to grow. How I had always enjoyed them, been proud of them, wanted them to be admired under my sweaters. How I liked them being fondled and appreciated by men. What pleasure I had nursing my three children, rocking and being suckled by their small mouths, while their small hands patted my breast. Surely there is no sweetness like that one, watching your babies grow, the milk from your breast trickling from the corners of their mouths as they fall asleep. And all of that is in the past. Warm in the late afternoon sun, I fondle my remaining breast, my flat half-chest, my armpit, my forearm. I let the flat of my hand rest against my scar. From a distance it would look as if I were making a vow. Then I pick up my notebook and begin to write.

Marilyn Hacker

❧

Journal Entries

Paris, November 23, 1992

A WEEK, AND THEN IT'S GONE, AND KJ TOO, AND now there's another week for me, as if the first one hadn't been. The "holiday" aspect of KJ's days here kept me away from this notebook. Now she's on her way to a surgery rotation in Oklahoma City—part of her mid-life transformation from a feminist bookseller to a physician assistant [the mid-level general practice profession that began with Vietnam-trained medics who weren't nurses] who'll work with AIDS patients. Where's the center I need to find for myself? We get better at comings and goings, though.

Tuesday evening, we went to Geneviève's for dinner. Wednesday: the Musée d'Orsay in the rain; dinner with Gail at Fandango in the evening. Thursday I (alone) walked down the rue du Faubourg St-Antoine to have a long lunch with Anne in her new place on the rue de Montreuil, with a terrace on the courtyard *and* windows on the street: later I met KJ for a (meretricious in my view; very popular) film, *Les Nuits Fauves:* bisexual AIDS as melodrama. Afterwards we walked across the river to eat at the Antillais place on rue Cardinal Lemoine. Friday the South American show at the Beaubourg; then I met Claire at "La Fourmi Ailée" for tea, looked over her Walcott translation. That evening, KJ and I went out in rain and métro strike to have dinner with Marie-Geneviève and Catherine, who hadn't met her yet.

KJ, looking good, handsome and slender and bilingually shy, was liked right off by both—and flirted with by M-G, who gave her a hand massage (her own hands pretty sexy work-callused with that missing finger-joint). Catherine has gone beyond *soupe au pistou*, which she used to brag was all she could cook, and produced a *navarin d'agneau*. A night for beaujolais nouveau, *saison oblige*. Marie-Geneviève, elfin and gravel-voiced, was pleased about new work included in a show of computer-palette art at the Palais de Japon. (I think her "*infographies*" will be impressive *Kenyon Review* covers.)

Somewhere in all that, KJ and I managed to make love three or four times. (The bad taste of "*Madame-combien-de-fois*"—but these days, with all our separations, it's how many times in two months, to happen in ten days.) Thursday night, one of those "*combien de fois*," Eleanor Bender [former editor of *Open Places*] called me from California, at 11:30 P.M. here, to tell me/us that Audre Lorde had died. We were in the high middle of sex; I initially sounded put out (Eleanor was surprised I'd be "asleep" at 11:30) until I heard the reason for the call. There was a profound echo of what happened seven years ago, in May 1985, when I was in bed with R one sunny and slightly hungover morning, and the phone rang. Who would it have been? I don't think it was KJ herself, who was too close, too shattered—but someone told me Sonny Wainwright, KJ's ex-lover and still closest friend, was in her final coma, and I should come and say good-bye. I didn't tell KJ that, last week. But the same thing happened we talked and held each other, and went back to, or forward with, our lovemaking, but in a different key.

KJ (and KJ with Sonny, as a couple) knew Audre the woman, as I had not. I only knew Audre the writer, Audre the activist, Audre the icon, from afar: Audre whose standards I, as a white feminist editor, sometimes failed to meet. I knew Audre most intimately through her books. Audre, as every one of her personae, will leave an unfillable gap. What can I do, here, now? Read poems?

I had a letter from R, who has had a "good MacDowell": nine new poems in various stages, one subtly slant-rhymed fourteen-liner in couplets, which is, for lack of an adequate word, "lovely." I replied with a long letter that was not much more than desultory: KJ's week here; *Kenyon Review* update: that the magazine is apparently getting a Lannan grant, with stated appreciation of its "multicultural content" which I worked my butt off to achieve; that *someone* told *someone* that President-elect Clinton said he would relax pre-inauguration by reading—an American President who reads!—among other things, "new African American writers in the *Kenyon Review.*"

Paris, November 26, 1992

Thanksgiving in the U.S.: should I revise my menu and cook poultry this evening for Marie-Geneviève and Catherine? I've been to market: diminished Thursday mornings, compared to Sunday (or late spring), but there are still three or four cheese-sellers and fishmongers, the North African greengrocers are out in near-full force, the biggest poultry-butcher's there (but not the mushroom stand). Jeweled piles of winter fruit: oranges, pineapples, clementines, apples. No pears—is it too late for pears?

The young woman of the student-looking couple across the way has her hair in braids today, down the front of a white smock. Sitting at the kitchen table, she looks like a Chinese schoolgirl. But—she also looks pregnant!

A long conversation with Rose [KJ's mom] from Florida. It took *sixteen hours* for KJ to get from New York to Oklahoma City: Midwestern blizzard, missed connections, airport delays—and still she was at work, beginning her surgery rotation, the next day (yesterday). How hard it is for me to imagine from this distance, so much further away than if she were in New York. And how difficult and strange it must be for her, plunged into an alien landscape, stalled in snow, with American Midwesterners (more foreign than Parisians or Dominicanos), to spend a month working *and* living in a hospital that's not even familiar Harlem. When we're in the same place, our lives intersect: we observe and interpret each other's experiences; we alternate who's sustaining whom. Then we're apart: increasingly, KJ's in the midst of situations which, if I can imagine them at all, are flattened, distorted by ignorance: I could be imagining a scene in a novel instead of a real operating room in Oklahoma City. Although she's seen it, "Gambier, Ohio" is still foreign to *her*, but my work there is familiar.

Books on my worktable: does James Wright flirt with sentimentality in a way Jack Spicer didn't, or is Spicer guarded in a way Wright didn't have to be? (Spicer as homosexual Jansenist.) Or—is Spicer's tough-guy obliquity another kind of sentimentality?

Paris, November 27, 1992

Another *grande bouffe* last night with Marie-Geneviève and Catherine. (It's still odd to see lone-wolf, more accurately Alpha-wolf Catherine—at the journal *Lesbia* anyway—let Marie-Geneviève lead their pack-of-two: not because she's twenty-seven years older, but by sheer force of personality.) They got here closer to 8:30 than 8:00: C in very wide-wale men's brown cords and a winter-sports polo-neck sweater; M-G in *red* baggy cords and black patent leather bovver boots! M-G brought the slide I want to use for the *KR* theater issue cover. I resisted the temptation to run Jean's translations of some poems by them: but she'll see them if she's to do a frontispiece. I'll enjoy sending her poems (French versions) as I've been able to see and appreciate so much of her own work.

M-G said how much she liked KJ. Catherine said she'd heard nothing *but* how much M-G had admired KJ since that evening! "But *you're* the most attractive," said M-G to C, cuffing her ears. I look forward to telling KJ she'd made an impression. The *lapin aux pleurottes* was a good idea. And the Savigny-les-Beaune rouge. Beaujolais nouveau loses its novelty, even in November (and I suppose I was secretly celebrating).

KJ called around 11, while we were finishing dinner—from a

phone booth in Oklahoma, to be the first (and only one so far) to wish me a happy birthday. I didn't mention the event to Marie-Geneviève, Catherine, Geneviève Pastre, the Migrennes... Still, I hoped for something in the mailbox this morning, which there wasn't. But Mme. Melhing was coming back from grocery shopping at 10 A.M., and asked me to carry her bag upstairs for her, with her daily baguette and pint of milk (not a bottle of wine; that was my own invention). As usual, she didn't recognize me, and asked what floor I lived on; as usual, I said I lived next door to her on the third. She thanked me with formal and exquisite politeness, and I responded that it was a pleasure to be of service to her... I hope it is a good omen for a fiftieth birthday to help a 102-year-old woman carry her groceries upstairs.

Yesterday went so swiftly; today's the same. Sometimes in Gambier, it seems like twelve hours between the *Kenyon Review* mail arriving at 10:30 and 3 P.M. as a mid-afternoon tea break (when I still usually have at least four office hours ahead of me). Why do I never want to go back to the apartment in Ohio, sit at the desk there, and look out at the trees with (sometimes) the sun setting behind them? Wouldn't that do as well as the roof of 26/Turenne and the neighbors across the way? Is what I should do here write down what I don't write down there: issues of the *KR* in progress; Nadine, the crusty librarian, gardening around her cabin shared by eighteen rescued stray cats. The personal/personnel dramas at the office are just what I want to be distanced from by an ocean.

Nowhere at all on this street was I when history-as-catastrophe (not as the daily graying and wearing of stone, the accumulation of mineral plaque in the pipes) happened. Did anyone knock on (fifty-two-year-old) Mme. Melhing's door in July 1942? Did a Jewish family, a Jewish widow or student, live where I live now, or upstairs, or downstairs where the Brescs took over two studio flats to break down walls and enlarge their five rooms in the adjacent building?

New York, January 4, 1993

Notebook/a line across a page or underneath a paragraph, more than a month or a year-date changed. I have lost a breast and a metaphor, a breast with cancer in it and a defective metaphor. I can no longer write poems in which the word "cancer" coldly and simply (and simple-mindedly) presages/stands in for "death." I intend (I bluster) to live, but I am (of course) scared shitless—as I said to the anesthesiologist before the drugs took effect. I've been falling off a cliff since Christmas Eve, though I hope I'm now standing at the bottom, on firm dry earth again. Now what?

On December 24 , having come in from Ohio with the tail end of a hangover, I went to Beekman Hospital for a routine mammogram; was scheduled to see Joan Waitkewicz later for an equally routine physical exam and Pap smear. After Audre's death, after Alicia Ostriker's recent story, I was, for the first time, frightened in the grubby little dressing-room, half naked, waiting for the x-ray tech to return. And she returned saying the radiologist had requested a second film of my right breast. Back to the machine, the painful compression and squeezing, another five minutes in limbo. KJ was sitting outside in the waiting-room with several Chinese families and a pregnant Latina teenager. For almost a month, our schedules had kept us apart: me in Paris, giving a reading in Milwaukee, back at the *Kenyon Review* in Ohio, and she on surgical rotation in Oklahoma City: we'd have made time to do the most banal errand together. And shaken by Audre's death, which in turn brought back Sonny's, this procedure didn't seem so banal to either of us. But then the radiologist, via the tech, gave the green light: it's OK, you can go.

So it was after that, after KJ and I drank cappuccino and chicken soup (respectively) in "Ellen's Starlite Diner," that, like an act of violence built up to in a suspense film, Joan Waitkewicz, in the course of her exam (KJ, in student mode, had just asked her: after you've done a routine breast exam, how do you teach the patient to do self-examination?), found a mass in my right breast. As far as any of us knew, it had not been there when she'd examined me a year earlier; neither KJ nor I had been aware of it when we were making love a few weeks ago, in bed on the rue de Turenne, or in bed at 105th Street the night before, when she had stroked and sucked my breasts—or when I was lathering myself in the shower, or lying alone in bed in Ohio, feeling my own breasts in tentative and terrified self-examination: what would I have done if I'd found a lump in my breast in the middle of the night in Ohio?

But it was Dr. Joan who found it, not in Ohio, but in New York, at four in the afternoon of Christmas Eve, with KJ there—who'd often herself been the patient, who had this time come with me for something "routine."

What good is repeating the melodrama of the following three-day weekend which I've replayed to a dozen well-wishers: Christmas Eve dinner at Santerello's with KJ *quand même;* queue-ing with the holiday throngs at Zabar's on Christmas afternoon for that evening's dinner here with Joan Schenkar, Anne Shaver, and Anne's partner, Susanne Wood; Iva on Saturday, Julie and Henry on Sunday evening. I told Joan, Iva [*my daughter*], Julie, not inclined to the masochism of keeping it to my/ourselves. And I/we still hoped for the release/reprieve: liquid cyst, fibroadenoma: bad scare, after which normal life resumes, with more awareness.

Monday we phoned breast surgeons. Dr. Joan had called three from her office, but it was late afternoon on Christmas Eve: she'd left "urgent" messages, with my phone number to be called back. KJ and I called eight, including the woman who'd performed Alicia Ostriker's mastectomy two years ago (a poem was dedicated to her in Alicia's sequence, which I'd published). Receptionists, answering machines told us when they'd be back from vacations, one possible appointment for mid-January.

And then we reached one man on a fluke, at the Strang Clinic at New York Hospital, Dr. William Curry, who was filling in for the vacationing chief of service. We bypassed the secretary's "He's not seeing anyone this week," with a wrong-headed question about a piece of diagnostic apparatus. Somehow this got us put directly through to Dr. Curry, who was actually in his office. And he made an appointment for the next morning.

KJ and I went down to Joan's office to collect the mammogram plates which we'd been asked to bring. The radiologist had seen exactly nothing in my "young," dense breast. I felt irrationally relieved, enough to go with KJ to get a haircut on Twenty-third Street, to stop at the Union Square market, to debate going to a film instead of home...

I saw Dr. Curry on Tuesday morning; he scheduled me for an excision biopsy at New York Hospital the next day. I fixated on the definition/diagram of "fibroadenoma" in the fairly simple-minded pamphlet he gave us; convinced myself he was implying that was what he thought it was. (William Curry was a courteous and handsome middle-aged [my age] African American. KJ's friend H, a breast cancer activist, had his name in her reams of information about good surgeons, but her connection with him was more personal—she remembered him as one of the few black students at her Great Neck high school.)

On Wednesday I was back at New York Hospital. "How are you feeling?" the burly red-headed anesthesiologist asked before he gave me the shot. "Scared shitless," I replied.

I awoke from the "twilight sleep" of the excision biopsy to be told by Dr. Curry that it was an invasive cancer; that he was admitting me and scheduling me for a mastectomy the next day—"If you were my sister, that's what I'd advise you to do." (I wondered, through my strangely flattened fear, if male surgeons are instructed to say "sister" in these cases, to imply "one of my own" without the, well, *transference* they'd be risking if they said "wife" or "daughter." And I imagined him as a brother.)

He was half kneeling beside me, where I was semi-reclined in one of the armchairs in the ambulatory-surgery recovery room, where the nervous bathrobed souls I'd seen in the admitting lounge downstairs were waking up, taking their juice and saltines, getting ready to go home. The elderly Orthodox Jewish woman accompanied by her frosted-blonde matron daughter had had a cataract removed; the tousled tweedy Irish-looking man I'd imagined was a journalist or newscaster was leaving with a redheaded wife and bored teenage daughter. KJ was with me. But I wasn't going home.

I instantly asked Dr. Curry if KJ could stay with me if I got a private room. "I'll have to kiss some nurses," he replied. I was moved into an empty, dark room adjacent to the recovery room to wait in what seemed like purgatory, despite KJ's presence. But by the time the room was ready upstairs, a cot had already been wheeled in for her. Joan S and Ellen both came by that evening (when I had hoped to be at home with KJ celebrating my reprieve). Under the bandage (from the biopsy, the lump's removal) on my chest was my right breast which I would never see again, the nipple, the mole above the nipple, whatever it had felt, or rather, what I had felt through it.

Yes, it was civilized for a hospital.

On the morning of New Year's Eve, Dr. Curry performed a modified radical mastectomy, removing, as well, some of my pectoralis minor and nearly all the lymph glands in my right armpit—forty of them.

Before the surgery, I'd talked to Iva; Chip [her father, novelist Samuel R. Delany]; Marie [Ponsot]; KJ's mom, Rose; a dozen other friends (some, like Alicia, with their own cancer stories); Y, the managing editor at the *Kenyon Review.* Just before the orderly strapped me to my mattress and winched it onto the gurney, I asked KJ to call R, feeling odd that this was the last thing I was asking her to do.

KJ was with me all those three days and nights—she herself only a few days back from her bizarre surgery rotation in Oklahoma City, where she'd spent weeks sleeping in an unused hospital room. Now she was sleeping in a hospital room again. We tried to share my bed the pre-op night, but it was too small for us with my discomfort from the biopsy. A nurse came in wake-you-up-to-see-if-you're-asleep rounds and ordered her back into her cot.

And those new words, new metaphors? The terrible lines I wake up with in the middle of the night are ones I've written myself: the lethal transformations of the breast, the deaths, and then again the deaths, of cancer. Let me write another book, let me face down the elegies a different way. Right now, when I read those poems, they seem like an affront to women and men who *have* had cancer, who are alive with their scars, with their nightmares, with their courage, with whatever else I don't know, or don't know yet. Another set of mastectomy poems, chemotherapy (if necessary) poems, can't you all be quiet?

(KJ says I should seriously consider having chemotherapy, even if the doctors don't insist on it, as a prophylaxis. I know she's thinking of Sonny, who didn't have it when she first had breast cancer— might it have prevented the metastasis that killed her ten years later?)

"How are you feeling? " asked the anesthesiologist again. "Still scared shitless." Dr. Curry sat next to me on a wooden stool (the now-familiar hydra-headed O.R. lights above my head) until— "I'm not asleep yet," and I was asleep. And then, without a paragraph break, I was back on the gurney in the in-patient surgical recovery room, Dr. Curry in my direct line of vision.

"It's all over. You're cured."

Paris, July 1995

I read this, and notice what, on my second day home from the hospital, I didn't write. Dr. Curry had kissed some more nurses to allow KJ, suited up like O.R. staff, to meet me when I woke up in the recovery room—*and* R, who had rushed there when she got KJ's call, and came in when KJ left (and brought an extravagant bouquet of big pink roses, which I found when I was taken upstairs to my room). Later in the day, Iva came, and Marie, and Charlie. Ellen came back that evening: she and KJ went out to find a deli in the not-promising Upper (far) East Side. I ate a few spoonfuls of whitefish salad that New Year's Eve after the liquid post-op hospital-hour dinner. The next morning, KJ went home and brought me back gray jersey pajama bottoms and a long-sleeved turquoise African-print T-shirt in which I was walking around the floor, pushing my I.V. pole, when Joan S came to visit with a New Year's Eve hangover. I slipped her some private-stock ibuprofen. Even when the morphine wore off, I couldn't dignify the pinchy, achy discomfort I felt with the name of "pain." I was only taking Tylenol 2 by the afternoon of January 1.

Dr. Curry came in to see me—in velour sweats, with his wife and sons waiting in the car downstairs to go to a New Year's Day basketball game. He examined his work with satisfaction—the first time I saw what was under the dressing. "Surgical staples" isn't a brisk, professional name for some kind of advanced plastic wound-sealer: I had metal staples like those I'd used on grade-school book reports from my sternum to my armpit. In the adjacent bathroom, Dr. Curry himself washed the yellow surgical disinfectant from my back, and showed me how to empty the plastic bulb-drain (like the bulb of a turkey baster) hanging from an opening: a small slash between my ribs: stigmata—and measure the liquid in it. Thus I didn't have to wait for the drain to be removed to be discharged. I went home the next day.

There'd also been the expected visit from the oncology nurse, Amy Chu, who came with a portfolio of frayed photographs of former patients five, ten years on: on a sailboat, with a small child and a new baby, playing with a collie. This routine to induce optimism only made me think of the photos she didn't have and would never show, and my own mental snapshots: Catherine Arthur bursting into terrified sobs in Compendium Bookshop after an uplifting chat with Patricia Duncker (herself now an eight-year cancer survivor) eighteen months before Catherine died; Sonny, vibrant in her bed at Mount Sinai, cheering and chatting with everyone who came with books, food, and flowers, as if her hospital bed were a café table—and Sonny not so long afterwards, on a respirator that she never wanted, in a coma, the rasp of her breath through the tube the only sound in the room.

I have only the vaguest recollection of Amy Chu's presentation of the "mastectomy bra" and its padded insert, a.k.a. "prosthesis" (as if it were a functional limb being replaced functionally—do they call it that when drag queens wear falsies?). I said I didn't plan to wear one, and don't clearly recall the conversation that followed. KJ says it was more or less urged on me: I might "change my mind when the weather got warm and I wanted to wear T-shirts." I believe I said that I'd want my half-flat-chested survivor status to be visible. Perhaps because this was so small an issue in my mind, perhaps because this conversation, since Audre's *Cancer Journals*, has almost become a literary trope, I've blocked it out. (A French friend, Jacqueline Julien, big-boned and small-breasted, was told by her woman oncologist that if she didn't plan to wear a false breast she might as well have the remaining one cut off!) But Amy Chu also brought an amateurishly illustrated exercise instruction booklet, which I would follow faithfully, daily, for the next six months, even adding small weights, until I may have been more limber than I was before.

Why the rush to surgery? I know now that the wide-margin excision biopsy had, in fact, extirpated the localized cancer from my body. This could have been made clear to me: perhaps, then, the night before the mastectomy, at least, wouldn't have been spent in such terror. I believe I would have made the choice I did any-way—and a ten days' wait before the mastectomy would not have improved my quality of life, nor that of those around me. This has never been, for me, about losing a breast

New York, January 6, 1993

The lymph node results were good: 100 percent clean, Dr. Curry said. That was yesterday afternoon, and today, with the drain out, I'm as depressed as I've been since this started. KJ is gone to start her E.R. rotation at Lincoln Hospital. Yesterday, when we got home from the doctor's, she broke down, revolted against all this for the first time. It would probably be better, she said, for her to go back and stay in her studio on 99th Street: she'd rather be there; the subway to Lincoln Hospital is more convenient.

It's my first day without her, spending the day alone: it's the first day since this began I've spent without being the center of somebody's attention: it's difficult. The dressing is off, so I'm aware how much (all) of the tightness and numbness and creepy-prickling-under-the-skin is caused by the incision/ablation, not by adhesive tape or a surgical bra too tight in the armpits. I read (reread, with a different perspective) Edith Konecky's novel, *A Place at the Table*, which R brought to the hospital. (They were Scrabble buddies at MacDowell.) It takes the reader by surprise with a breast-cancer chapter at the end, which is written, more of a surprise, with wry humor.

I finished Toni Morrison's *Jazz*, which I began in the hospital, noting that she and Chip had both picked the year 1924 in Harlem as a setting, an organizing principle, for a work of fiction. My other hospital reading had been Donald Hall's *Their Ancient, Glittering Eyes*, a book of reminiscences of poets, mostly old, distinguished poets. I needed to read about old poets. Here, I have Hall's *The Museum of Clear Ideas*, poems which include the discovery of a "quiet carcinoma" in his colon.

Iva and KJ both came with me to Dr. Curry's office yesterday afternoon. He had been in surgery all morning, was late for my appointment, but called his secretary to say he was on his way, and to tell us that, though he couldn't give us details on the phone, it was good news.(No cancer cells in the dissected lymph nodes!)

KJ and Iva both came into the examination room with me. I stripped off sweater and black T-shirt; he took off the surgical bra and the dressing, and examined the enormous scar, toothed with metal staples, which goes up into my armpit, then clipped the stitch in my side and took out the plastic drain-tube and bulb. I was glad Iva watched: she wouldn't have to wonder what it looked like, fear some unknown horror: it looks as extreme now as it ever will.

Konecky's chapter ends with the protagonist and her eighty-four-year-old mother watching a white "Mediwaste" truck going down Second Avenue (from New York Hospital, where we both had our surgery): disposal of tainted, rebellious body parts. In the next chapter, she's riding alone on the subway, with a notebook. No falsies: she's put fountain pens in her left breast pocket, searched for shirts which *had* left breast pockets (Right, in my case, and harder to find!) Her protagonist is told by the doctors, "You *had* cancer, it's over. Now go and live your life." Is that what Dr. Curry said to me? Would I have believed him?

Stay in Ohio for six months of chemotherapy, through the long winter? Would that mean a long slow drive twice a month back and forth from Columbus, with the slightly retarded Church of the Nazarene driver picking his teeth? The two/three monthly days of sickness and exhaustion leaving me dependent on the kindness of (after two years) virtual strangers in Gambier? I'm getting this ass-backwards. To not get it ass-backwards (with post-operative con-stipation to boot), I must envision a positive goal, however New Agey that sounds: to live and appreciate my life, to get limber and get well, to use living and appreciating my life as a means of get-ting/staying well.

New York, January 8, 1993

Late morning, gray day. KJ's at Lincoln Hospital. We haven't talked any more about her moving back to 99th Street: she's con-tinued to stay here with me, to my enormous relief. I'm waiting for a call-back from Dr. Curry. I'm seeing oncologist #1 this after-noon: Dr. Curry's referral and recommendation. Longish talk with Judy Moffett; a check-in from the surgical oncology nurse, Amy Chu.

Paris, July 1995

Judith Moffett, poet and science fiction novelist whom I first met at MacDowell in 1978, had, in 1993, recently passed the five-years-clean mark after a breast cancer I took very seriously indeed: six invaded lymph nodes. She had CAF (Adriamycin) chemotherapy, which knocked her flat. A year later, she and her twenty-years-older medievalist spouse turned their Pennsylvania acre into a survival garden—a "homestead," where they raised all the food they ate, including fish, ducks, honey from their own beehives (this last despite the threat of lymphedema from bee stings in the arm whose lymph nodes were removed: it didn't happen). Just the idea of this enterprise felt curative to me, who'll never come any closer to it that reading the book Judy wrote about it.

She had become, before the cancer diagnosis, adept at Transcendental Meditation, good enough to heal a wart on her foot by concentration/visualization—which she said helped her through both the chemotherapy and the panic; she strongly recommended the books on visualization that KJ had unearthed from her own periods of dealing with illness.

Judy was a long-distance mentor to me all through the next six months: she'd been to a worse place; she'd educated herself and taken charge; she also had acknowledged her terror, her realization that the combat was mortal. And we had a lot in common besides breast cancer (metered poetry, science fiction in my past and her present) which enabled us to decompress in those long-distance conversations: our connection wasn't defined by a disease.

New York, January 14, 1993

Iva's nineteenth birthday—and two weeks since the surgery. I've had up and down days: today could be a downer if I don't watch out. I wish I were a writer with a project. Edmund [White] has finished his Genet biography, and is overjoyed to be writing fiction again. I have a new notebook to follow this notebook, by whose final pages I have left the "country of ordinary, snub-nosed mortals" (Auden) who have not come up against cancer or HIV, against something that makes prolonged survival moot, one's whole life and its purposes and occupations something to be reflected upon and reconsidered. Edmund left that "ordinary" company in 1985 when he tested positive. KJ, or anyone vaguely Buddhist, would say, in so many words, that life is everywhere precarious—bluntly, that anyone can drop dead anytime.

"Cancer is a disease of animals; canker is a disease of plants"— Stephen Dedalus memorizes that in *Portrait of the Artist*... Despair the canker (cancer) of the (flowering) spirit?

The first oncologist, Dr. G, was a puppy, a dark-haired boy (in his thirties) who kept us waiting forty-five minutes beyond the appointment time, when KJ had left her own clinic early to meet me there. Iva came with me from home. He sat, enthroned behind an enormous mahogany desk, the three of us crowded on the other side; then had us meet his chemotherapy nurse in the treatment room, a platinum blonde with a Russian accent, who asked me what had been wrong with me. It seemed an odd question in that office; then I realized she wanted me to pronounce the name of the disease, to show I wasn't denying it. "I had an infiltrative ductal carcinoma, one cm in size, with a microscopic secondary tumor, but no lymph node involvement detected." (Iva, unusually outspoken, said on the way home that she'd be surprised and upset if I decided to be treated by Dr. G. No one disagreed with her.)

The second oncologist, Anne Moore, whom I saw this past Tuesday, is a tall blonde woman about my age. All three of us felt more confident and comfortable with her—beginning when she seated us *with* her at a medium-sized round wooden table. The two doctors' recommendations were the same, though: a six-month course of CMF chemotherapy, possibly to be done back and forth between New York and Ohio, where Dr. Moore has colleagues: an oncologist from Columbus is now also connected to the hospital in Mount Vernon (five miles from Kenyon College instead of forty-five). Yes, there were colleagues she knew in Paris. The two best pieces of news I'd had that day.

I'm in a tailspin today, mind adjunct to body—I kept myself from writing "my betraying body." But there's no "me" and "it": mind/body. I'm the sum of my parts. I think of blighted plants keeling over, uprooted and tossed on the compost heap. But the blight (the surgeon said) has been excised.

I've canceled the New Mexico reading, canceled the Colgate reading, canceled the California readings for the beginning of May, called Jean Migrenne and told him, said I wouldn't be able to come and talk to his students in Caen later in May. It was as if I was canceling everything to which I might look forward in the next four months. I exaggerate. But I've been writing letters, making phone calls, "announcing" my condition to the world: Bill in San Francisco, Lilian Mohin in London, Marie-Geneviève and Catherine, Edmund and Hubert, Gail in Paris. Geneviève's sister died of breast cancer; Odile's sister-in-law is dying of metastasized breast cancer, which makes me reluctant to call or write to each of them. But I want "everyone" to know—as if their affection and good wishes would keep me safe. And closer to them all.

Four-thirty or so. Alfred Corn was here for tea, early, on his way up to Columbia for a beginning-of-term sherry party. Jane Cooper came yesterday. She'd asked what she could bring: why, things for tea. So she arrived with a small orange-walnut loaf and miniature chocolate cupcakes—and a group of her own new poems, mostly from her recent MacDowell residence, which I read while she was here. Despite some disconsolate book-chat— no obvious publisher for her new collection, as she's, unreasonably, not part of any easily published in-group, a feeling of accomplishment and satisfaction. Jane with gray page-boy, plum-colored plaid mohair skirt, some soft peach turtleneck I hope was cashmere, with a remarkable batch of new poems, new energy, in her seventieth year.

Deaths of women by cancer; love as a chant against death—the last thing I wrote, go beyond it, to survival, cancer not as the unknown but certain doom, but the trial I'm living through, a way to understand more than I did before, to be able to ask, with more comprehension, Simone Weil's question: "What are you going through?"

Even Adrienne, the poet perhaps most focused on our collective survival, wrote "A Woman Dead in Her Forties," another bleak elegy for someone killed by breast cancer. Has she, yet, written about someone living with it/through it/past it—Audre, when she was alive? She has, though, written about her own disease, her own literal coexistence with pain, and written "out" from there—perhaps the most any of us can do honestly.

Paris, July 1995

Though not specifically about "cancer," Adrienne Rich *had* written a powerful poem precisely on the speciousness of a division between "victims" and "survivors," since we are both at once, "From Corralitos Under Rolls of Cloud," in *An Atlas of the Difficult World*, which I had read in galleys in Paris in May of 1991, a book I have in both my cities:

> What does it mean to say I have survived
> until you take the mirrors and turn them outward
> and read your own face in their outraged light?

And Alicia Ostriker's sequence of "Mastectomy Poems," which I'd read in manuscript, and of which I'd taken a group of five for publication in the *Kenyon Review*, is vividly about a woman living through and after breast cancer, and embodies her refusal to be diminished to the "victim" role, while chronicling her fear and loss. I *was* depressed, and depression engenders solipsism.

New York, January 26, 1993

Evening, or twilight: "teatime," a quarter after five. Mostly a good day, in which I read a box of manuscripts for the *Kenyon*

Review, and set up a development consultancy for Eleanor Bender at Kenyon the week of February 27; she'll arrive in Gambier the day after what should be the second round of my second chemo treatment.

Iva left for school a week ago Saturday—the sixteenth—in a car with three other young women. One of them, a handsome brunette called Wendy, had been in my office in November on behalf of the Latino students' group to discuss jointly bringing Martín Espada to Kenyon for a reading: she's also a Bronx Science grad. KJ had worked in the E.R. that day, in order to have Monday off, so we could go together to Audre's memorial service at St. John's. I'd spent the morning "perfecting" *Kenyon Review* direct-mail subscription letters: part of the Lila Wallace marketing grant. Living with Iva (again) was a palliative in those two-weeks-after-surgery. I've missed her since.

Dr. Curry took the last staples out last Thursday, after which I walked the couple of blocks to New York Hospital for a briefing with the oncology nurse, Marta, a compact, brown-skinned Panamanian (she told me, and about her teacher brother and baby son) woman whom I liked and trusted on meeting. Edith Konecky met me in the waiting room. I had called her to say how much I'd appreciated *A Place at the Table*, and we'd made this date, in a place she knows well, as we are both now lifetime patients of Anne Moore's. We went to lunch across First Avenue; I gave her a copy of *Going Back to the River.*

Friday morning I went back to the hospital for the first chemotherapy treatment. Marie met me there. I'd worn a denim workshirt with buttons in front and sleeves I can roll up, so I wouldn't have to wear a hospital gown for the procedure: I didn't know how long it would take; my own clothes made me feel more in control. Waiting for the doctor, I took off the shirt, and my undershirt, and put the shirt back on, open, over my bare chest. Dr. Moore examined my apparently well-healing scar, which every-one medical "admires"—likewise my arm mobility, which I've worked on daily. (Much easier, of course, to approach this disease

as if it were my recovery from a traumatic motorcycle crackup.)
Then Marie came into the treatment room with me. I took an anti-
nausea pill; Dr. Moore herself inserted the butterfly needle quickly,
drew a vial of blood, then attached two syringes of medication, all
in and out the same minuscule needle: that was it.

No drama, no side effects (yet). Marie took me home in a cab.
I made tea; she stayed, and we talked until KJ came home at four.
Marie planned to rent my Paris apartment for a stretch this win-
ter/spring. Then (despite "retirement"), she was invited for three
university consultancies in early February, and a well-paid one-
month semester workshop in April. So she'll be on the rue de
Turenne from February 18 through March. The next-best thing to
my being there.

This morning I called Odile in Paris and told her. Our last conversation—over dinner in November in the rue Princesse—had
been about cancer fatalities: her school friend, her sister-in-law.
This time, she talked about her eighty-three-year-old mother, who
had breast cancer twelve years ago; her grandmother, who had it at
thirty, and lived forty-six years after that. Not the Résistance
grandmother—that would have been perfect. She'd like Marie to
read at the bookshop in my place in March: I could do something
in late June, even early July, before the August absences begin.

All the self-help books (which KJ retrieved from her bookshelves, which Judy Moffett, and the social worker, and others, recommended) I read frighten me, between the descriptions of
debilitating chemotherapy side-effects, which I'm not yet experiencing, and those of advanced metastatic cancer cases, even when
the story's end is a remission through chemotherapy/diet/visual-
ization and meditation: what often sounds like "willpower."

I feel best, of course, when I'm not thinking about cancer, or
when I'm concentrating on the arm and shoulder exercises, as if I
had been in a car crash, as if the surgery had been, as Dr. Curry
called it, a "cure." Of course I want to "visualize" myself healthy,
finishing a new book, taking a long walk with KJ, writing at my

desk here or on the rue de Turenne, celebrating KJ's graduation with her in the late fall in Burgundy—her graduation, and the Christmas/New Year's holidays that will now always be the anniversary of the lump, the New Year's Eve surgery.

Instead come the mental tailspins: did Dr. Curry's optimistic statistics figure in women with microscopic cancers found almost by accident like Helen's or Marge's, or in mammography like Alicia's? What were the "statistics" for someone with an infiltrative carcinoma? The theory that I can influence the outcome is as terrifying as it is reassuring (a metastasis would be "my fault")—even though I'm fairly sure I "influenced" (positively) my experience of pregnancy and childbirth, quit smoking, acknowledged and assumed lesbian sexuality in my early thirties, not a passive process at all: from being an awkward, reluctant lover to a passionate one, to maintaining a day-to-month-to-year relationship without losing that passion...That idea of "influence"—as in the Simonton books— is also terrifying because I fall so neatly into their category of person-set-up-to-develop-cancer (how I "participated in my illness") with stress in the last twelve months: separations from KJ more and more prolonged; increasing pressure at work last spring with the Lila Wallace marathon marketing grant application; cutting my time in Paris short because of that, and not being "productive" there, coming back to the overwhelming Lila Wallace project, and Y's fury at my absence flaring up every time I "dared" to criticize the way she'd done, or not done, some grant-related thing, culminating with her resignation letter turned in to the provost over my head, a copy in my mail basket after the fact. Her prolonged, furious (and verbally inventive, take-no-prisoners) outbursts happened only three times between late July and early November, but each time, I felt as if I were, indeed, walking away from a car crash. And a year, a year and a half now, of practically "not writing"—four poems, a few translations, last summer's exercises in a notebook in my office in Ohio.

And "what was the hidden benefit" of my illness, or however the phrase goes? More than a month in New York living with KJ, doing what I can of my work for the *Kenyon Review* and getting a nightly update of hers (Lincoln Hospital E.R. in the Bronx this rotation). Living with Iva again. The attention given a "convalescent" and an "invalid" who's up to making conversation: all those loquacious teatimes with cakes and flowers. Had I "accomplished" this with a case of walking pneumonia or a broken leg, I might have counted it an even trade.

I hate being a predictable "case history." Instead of thinking that their system will therefore work for me, I scare myself with the mortal retribution that might follow if I don't adhere to/succeed with that system...

New York, January 30, 1993

5:45 P.M. Will I, please, may I, again be the person writing at the table facing the window in the rue de Turenne at dusk. Well then, right now I'm writing at the desk in my office on 105th Street at dusk, or just past, and KJ's resting in the bedroom: appreciate it.

The second chemo treatment (technically: the second part of the first one) went as uneventfully as the first, except that Marta the RN gave me the injections this time, and left a little scar in the crook of my arm that burns a bit. They said my bloods were good. Earlier, Dr. Curry had admired his handiwork again and removed a few strips of the surgical tape. I brought Dr. Moore a list of the vitamins and minerals I've started taking. But neither Dr. Moore nor Marta seemed particularly concerned about vitamin therapy and maintenance vitamins. "Just eat a lot of crunchy vegetables." (Which I've never *not* eaten, have been teased about the ubiquity of broccoli, collard greens, cabbage, salads on my non-vegetarian table. I love crunchy vegetables—didn't they love me back?)

Marie met me at the hospital again, read the *Times* in the waiting room this time while I had the treatment. We came across and uptown in a cab and shared duck liver mousse and eggplant terrine for lunch at Positively 104th Street. She said, à propos of "Against

Elegies"—which now seems like bleak prediction in a poem—that my perceptions were a bit skewed, because the people of her generation who were going to die in their thirties, forties, fifties, were already dead. But she added quickly, perhaps thinking of her five or six Queens College colleagues, closer to my age than hers, who had been killed by cancer, that the prevalence of cancer in my generation—not to mention the scourge of AIDS—was unprecedented, astounding. Later, I showed her the two prose poems Jane Cooper had sent me after our tea three weeks ago. Marie recounted a dream she'd had last week in which Jane had written a new long poem about another American literary figure (on the model of her Willa Cather poem) .

Let *me* (as I apostrophized in "Against Elegies") be sixty in ten years, and have ten healthy, work-filled years, years with KJ and my friends, between now and then. Let me be healthy at fifty-one, and have a few pages to show for it, that's what, a prayer? I woke up once in the night drenched with sweat, the incision aching—though I'd been sleeping soundly, no bad dreams, until then. A side effect, I suppose. *I'd* like to dream about gentle and generous septuagenarian poets writing new long poems.

New York, February 7, 1993

I slept all right. I had hoped KJ and I would feel close and energetic enough to make love this (Sunday) morning, but we didn't. (It's always difficult when it's the "last time for a while," all the more so now.) This is no time to ask her / ask myself, will we ever have a—what would be the word—normal? normally queer? regularly irregular sex life again? However I feel about having a foot-long scar where my right breast used to be, the few times we've made love since the hospital, I've felt renewed, energetic, better.

Sex is a meditation; writing is a meditation. Whether or not writing (sex?) is that place where there's, as Bill put it, "an island of mental relaxation," it is that place where, as long as it lasts, there is nothing other than itself, what I'm doing in that moment: I'm not obsessing on the lost past and questionable future. Keep doing it, then—writing, if not sex. Make time in Ohio, in those morning hours I'll eventually have.

I have no idea how I'll feel when I come back in mid-March after/during cycle three of chemo. I'm trying to think as positively as possible about what's waiting for me in Ohio. The best part will be, of course, the office desk piled up with manuscripts and correspondence, always some serendipitous surprises amidst the dross. Noon by the time I get there, after the drive from the Columbus airport—a few hours in the office, preliminary exploration of those piles, then back to the empty apartment, in whose fridge I hope Iva put some staples. (I'm not sure how I'll get back to the apartment from the office—about a half-mile—if there's snow and ice.)

Paris, July 1995

How blithely and (again) solipsistically I referred to "sex," as if I were trying to prove something to myself, or to an imaginary reader over my shoulder. The truth was not as blithe, and more predictably complex. I wanted to prove to myself (and my lover) that I was still sexual. Not that I was still attractive to her—she'd already fallen in love with a woman who'd had a double mastectomy: androgyny, even achieved by such radical means, has always attracted her at least as much as "high femme." No, I needed to prove to myself that *I* still had sexual desires, responses, could give and receive those particular pleasures, could concentrate on her body and be concentrated in my own. I wanted to *be* sexual more than I *felt* sexual: what I most wanted was to be held. And, more than once (in January, in February, and later) when we'd begin to make love, got to anything more complex or specific than kissing, when I was launched on the sometimes solitary-seeming trajectory to orgasm, the fantasies which would come, unbidden, in response to those very corporeal caresses were not erotic but morbid. Sexual arousal pulled me into my body, and my body had demonstrated its mortality. My own tumescence made me think of death.

This didn't make an already fraught situation—memory-fraught and fraught in the present moment—any easier for KJ. And I couldn't think of anyone with whom I could discuss what was happening. The most obvious interlocutors—Sonny, Catherine Arthur, Audre—were dead. (Sex was not something I'd ever talked about with Judy Moffett; June Jordan seemed, to me, anyway, to prefer not to talk about cancer.) Now I think I might have talked to Alicia Ostriker: although she's straight, although we're more mutually appreciative literary colleagues than close friends, breast cancer makes for a kind of instant sorority; she is eloquent and frank enough as a writer about both sexuality *and* cancer to make me think the subject could be broached in conversation. Solipsism and depression are only ingenious in self-perpetuation. Marianne Weil, Edith Konecky—I could have started a support group just among women I knew. KJ herself would have been someone to talk to—if we hadn't been lovers, if my problem hadn't also been hers.

Gambier, Ohio, February 9, 1993

7:30 A.M: I have half an hour before Nadine collects me. The sky's gelid gray, the roads are icy; I've barely made a dent in the piles on my office desk, but that was just my first day back. I got up at ten past six, made tea, ate half a grapefruit and half an English muffin with jam—I'll have lunch with Iva—did my exercises and followed the "white light" meditation tape. Is this a meditation, as I push away the clouds of disruptive thoughts? Peaceful island . . .

The English faculty had left a flower arrangement on the file cabinet in my broom-closet sized office—not on the desk, which was covered by four stacks and two wire baskets full of mail: letters, unsorted flyers, hundreds of manuscript envelopes (despite the three boxes of same sent to me which I'd dealt with in New York). And there was a little garden bunch in a glass vase from Y,

with a notecard saying "Good for one lunch at the Pine Tree Barn."
Yet, on the phone yesterday morning, in New York, minutes before
I left for the airport, she'd set me on edge by complaining about
the "time that would be lost from the new managing-editor interview process" because two people involved—myself and one other
staff member—would be going to the hospital on the morning of
February 19 for my chemotherapy. I was too stunned to respond.
I called her back, when I'd collected myself, to say that I had never
expected anyone from the *Kenyon Review* to go to the hospital with
me: I'd go with a friend, or Iva, or a hired student driver.

Paris, July 1995

A kind of abandonment, although I never said it, was what I
was experiencing. Perhaps, in the context of my illness, it was too
frightening to admit. In the two and a half years I'd been at the
Kenyon Review, Y's friendship, intelligence, wit, and good sense
had sustained me through the hothouse rivalries endemic to an
isolated small college. Y was a big, redheaded Irish woman my age,
raised on a farm some thirty miles from Gambier, where her
mother still lived. A devout but independent Catholic, she'd gone
to a Catholic women's college, taken an M.A. in journalism at the
state university, worked for ten years as an editor for the
Environmental Protection Agency in Washington, then married
and returned to Ohio, where she'd worked in local radio before
coming to the *Kenyon Review*. She kept herself apart from the
"professors," who showed (as far as I could see) little interest in
her, despite her experience, keen intelligence, and education. It
was as clear a class rift as I could imagine. Almost all the faculty
were, like me, from elsewhere: largely Episcopalian with a mostly
leftish Jewish minority. A rural working-class Irish Catholic was
much more alien to them than (for example) an Ivy League-edu-
cated African American—whom they'd have assiduously courted.
But Y didn't cultivate *them* either: her friendly gestures were for
the clerical and administrative staff; what she knew about libera-

tion theology, environmental policy, and Irish poetry, she kept to herself.

My librarian friend Nadine was similarly an outsider. Although she had a Ph.D. in the History of Science, and ten years' non-tenured teaching experience at a small women's college, she'd been hired at Kenyon as a librarian—her profession before the mid-life Ph.D. Like Y, she was working-class in upbringing (Minnesota Lutheran in her case) and identification. In her mid-sixties, a heart attack survivor, short, slightly lame, bookish, crotchety; she lived in a tumbledown rented cabin with a profuse garden and eighteen half-wild cats. At Kenyon, she was beyond the pale.

Y knew the Central Ohio countryside, its geographical quirks, beauties, history, the way a lover knows the face and childhood reminiscences of her beloved. She had taken me on long drives: to the (now tourist-ridden) Amish villages; the second-hand furniture store out of which I decorated my Gambier apartment; the quilt shop in Mount Vernon which sold local (non-Amish) women's inventive work.

She had (she said) never worked for a woman. She proudly called herself a feminist, and was scathing about my predecessors' abdications of responsibility (not answering their mail for eight months, inventing grandiose projects whose administrative details became *her* unpaid overtime responsibility). To her, they were both implicated and exonerated by the fact of being "professors." (The Lila Wallace marketing grant must have seemed like more of the same, a project she would not have chosen to undertake.) She was adamantly anti-abortion: wouldn't have an issue of *Ms.* in her home (I'd offered to pass along my subscription copies) because of its pro-choice activism. But she also deplored the papal ban on contraception, supported the ordination of women... *Ms.* aside, we shared books: Elizabeth Bowen, Nancy Mairs, Ernesto Cardenal. Sometimes, and only after asking if it was an imposition (and specifying "no rush"), I'd asked for her opinion on manuscripts about which I was uncertain—usually essays combining literary and social issues. The letters of commentary she returned were mordant, elegant, sometimes devastating (or they would have been, had the writer in question seen them). I'd expected the few scrawled-but-pertinent sentences I usually got from consulting editors: she'd hand me two or three typed pages of witty and acute critical prose.

Still, what I largely remember of the first two years we worked together is those long occasional jaunts after work in her fifteen-year-old banger to covered bridges, the Amish hardware store, the quilt shop, or to some hill between pastures we'd walk up and watch the sunset.

Gambier, Ohio, February 20, 1993

Early morning, late winter, but deep winter: low teens outside or worse, snow on the ground, ice on the road, more snow expected. A week since I've sat down with this notebook, even though I called it "a meditation."

My hair is falling out. This has been going on for, say, five days (before which I'd seen fewer hairs on my comb than I had last fall). Every morning I spend at least ten minutes just after getting out of bed, cleaning the loose hairs off my pajama shirt, the pillowcase, the sheet (with Scotch tape rolled around my fingers). If I run my hand through my hair, it comes out full of loose hairs, ditto my rather large-toothed comb. I knew this might happen—but I envisioned it later, in April, when getting a crew cut might seem seasonally appropriate.

I went to the local hospital last Friday (the twelfth) and my white blood count had plummeted. I was supposed to see the Columbus oncologist, Dr. Ungerleider, on his monthly visit to the Mount Vernon hospital this past Tuesday—but he didn't get there because of a snowstorm, and left orders that I wasn't to get the treatment yesterday. I got a lift in yesterday, anyway, for another blood test. They don't have instant results here, as at New York Hospital, but I called in later, and the white count was back up to 4. I was ready to walk the two miles back in the snow and have my shots, but the oncology nurse said I couldn't until I'd seen the doctor this coming Tuesday. I'd talked with Dr. Moore on the phone earlier (who concurred in the delay); I should have called her back with the improved white count, and asked her to contact Ungerleider, so I could at least be sure of having the treatment on Tuesday.

A week's delay: June 18 becomes June 25; and "normal life" recedes as well, whatever that will be. Will I always be aware of the long scar across my chest, the near-painful tightness in my armpit, the vulnerability of having so little muscle between my ribs and the world? I want it to be over: you had breast cancer; now you don't. I want to have productive decades like Hayden Carruth, Josephine Jacobsen, Marie (who arrived at my place in Paris this morning). Common sense says that "productive" starts today; otherwise I could live to be eighty-five, still waiting for another "golden season," a crown of sonnets in four days, the form or shape of some kind of poem I'd never envisioned before.

Rafael Campo wrote to me, and *did* include thirty-two sonnets, one sequence of sixteen which he'd written after his own cancer scare: a suspicious cyst on a bone in his arm that had been broken in a skiing accident when he was sixteen. (In the sonnets, he's only twenty-six—how old, how *young* is he now?) I wrote back to say I'd like to publish "Song Before Death" (which hasn't even been logged in at the office)—and that I was impressed and frankly envious: here's what he did with *his* fears, intern's schedule notwithstanding. What have I made of mine?

Hayden Carruth sent me: a letter describing his daughter Martha's ongoing struggle with metastasized liver cancer (she's a painter, she's working); his eminently readable essay collection, *Suicides and Jazzers*, and a new long poem called "The Camps," "about" Bosnia, Somalia, Chile, Auschwitz, our century (he'd been reading Charles Simic's translations of Yugoslavian poetry—now one has to ask: Serb, Croat, or Muslim—*o tempera o mores*). He wrote that two poet/critic friends had read it: one found it "too undigested," and the other "too surreal." I'm an inveterate blue-penciller of other people's poems, but I had no such impulse with this one; was only glad to be an editor when I read it. I wrote back that it was, in my humble opinion, fucking brilliant, that I wanted to publish it—and that he'd lost all right to bitch and moan that he'd "written himself out" at seventy-one.

I feel as if Rafael and Hayden, neither of whom I've ever met in person (and who don't know each other) have become my good friends, "blood brothers" in the art—an inestimable benefit of my position as editor here: in each case we "met" when they submitted poems (though I've been reading Hayden's work for years).

A paper napkin on the desk's now covered with loose, dark, oily hair—mine, and despite last night's shampoo—just from running my hand through it as I write. The hair loss is "trivial," transi-tory—after chemotherapy, it grows back. Judy Moffett said hers came back thicker, and curlier. But to so many observers, that sparse hair or shaved head means "cancer," they note it and think "someone marked for imminent death," as they might think seeing a Kaposi's lesion. It's that vision of myself seen as marked by "can-cer" (not by what's being done to prevent its recurrence) that makes the hair loss upsetting. Some of those ill-informed observers see the absence of hair as a *symptom* of cancer, not a side effect of treatment. (Make another cup of milky decaf tea, throw away the napkin full of hair into the bedside wastebasket, whose plastic liner's full of hair already.)

The thermostat says the house is warm, but I'm not. Because this isn't New York or Paris, because the roads are icy and the tem-perature glacial, I've hardly been out walking. I wish KJ were in the next room. I wish I were healthy and strong. I wish—for that mat-ter—it were sunny out, with a temperature of 45 degrees, so I could go for a walk.

Eleanor's protegée, Gretchen W, came last week to interview for the managing editor's job. This entailed: a meeting with me and the rest of the search committee, lunch alone with me, a morning with Y being shown the routines and equipment, separate meetings with five administrators, from president to treasurer; dinner with me and Laurie Finke, the new Women's Studies director—plus, last Saturday, a hike around the campus with me and Y to see Kenyon's "historic" buildings, and a drive to Mount Vernon's quilt shop.

Y came to pick me up to take Gretchen around campus: an exhausting walk in six inches of snow from one end of Middle Path to the other. I ran up and down the stairs in Pierce and Ascension Halls to show her the stained glass and woodwork which Y, with an arthritic knee that precludes stair-climbing, thought she should see. When she arrived, with Gretchen in tow, Y came into the kitchen and wiped her wet snow boots on the red wool hooked rug from the grandfatherly weaver's shop in Berlin, Ohio, in front of the stove. "Y, not on the rug!" I said, laughing. The day passed, Gretchen left for the airport. I came home and fell out, fully dressed, to be waked up by Y knocking on the door at ten to six, to go to the Black Students' Union annual soul-food dinner at Pierce Hall, of which Iva was one of the hosts. We were meeting Nadine there.

As soon as I was in the car and had closed the door, Y told me indignantly how deeply I'd insulted her by asking her not to wipe her boots on the rug. I'd made her feel "like a little dog." I'd never have known where to buy that rug without her. I was arrogant and inconsiderate and she wasn't the only one to think so! She didn't know if "all New York people were like that." And on nonstop until she'd parked the car. I felt (I know it sounds histrionic) beaten, battered: tired and overextended as I was, unexpected as this was. I thought we'd had a good afternoon with Gretchen; I thought Y might recall asking me to be the sightseeing guide up and down four flights of stairs in two buildings, despite chemo fatigue. It was like a childhood scene with my mother, who'd suggest a walk for what I thought would be companionate conversation, and instead, once we were alone, she'd yell at me for being fat lazy unathletic unpopular...

Nadine was waiting for us outside Pierce Lounge, in a new velvet brocade suit. Nothing for it but for me to sit with them, between them, for Nadine's sake (she said I was looking very pale). We sat down at a table opposite a black family from Columbus: mother, father, grandmother, younger brothers of a Kenyon sophomore—with whom I had to rouse myself from exhaustion and misery to make conversation. Iva was at the student hosts' table on a raised platform with the invited speaker, a bass-voiced Baptist clergyman who gave a fairly rousing address much later. I motioned to two English department women to take the empty seats at the other end of our table, but they sat with their spouses at another, all-faculty table, where I longed to go myself, away from Y, get a few "strokes" as a convalescent—but I couldn't, because of Nadine and the Columbus family.

We were seated at 6:15, and weren't "sent up" to get our food from the buffet until 7:30: that hour-and-a-quarter, without the distraction of food, speeches, or entertainment, was excruciating. I couldn't table-hop (no one was doing that); I was painfully aware of Y being gregariously charming to the Columbus family, and how I was failing in that respect. I wanted to sit with Iva. I wanted to go home and pull the comforter over my head.

The next morning, I had a bad headache that continued for two days.

The following Monday, Nadine (bless her) took me down to Mount Vernon again to pick up my prescriptions. She said that, in the cloakroom, she'd told Y I wasn't looking well, and Y had said she'd "given me a talking-to." She, Nadine, thought Y was focusing all her anger and dissatisfaction with her job, and the atmosphere at Kenyon, on me. But that getting to know me had been one of the best things to happen to *her* in Gambier. I felt better.

On Tuesday morning, in my office, I wrote a long letter to Y. Did she realize how deeply her anger affected me? Was she, perhaps, venting her eight years of Kenyon-related frustrations at me? How I valued her as a colleague, as a friend (though while I was writing the letter I never wanted to see her again). She took Wednesday off: it was her birthday and there was a snowstorm. She's been amicable ever since, as she usually is, after giving me hell. But she's made no reference to the letter.

Gambier, Ohio, February 21, 1993

Past 10 A.M.—but I got started earlier, even working on a couple of so-far so-so sonnets that I could envision becoming part of a "braided crown," about, what else, breast cancer and exile in Ohio. I exercised; I "did" my meditation tape; I spoke to Marie at (my) home in Paris, (7 A.M. my time; 1 P.M. hers), safe and warm but needing to be reminded how to turn on the hot water heater. I felt on solid ground in my own world talking to her. And when...? Live *now*. Sunday, February 21, going on 11 A.M., Bach flute/recorder concerto playing and, yes, my hair falling out, and my right armpit feels as if it has staples in it still. A half-dozen more *KR* manuscripts read. I could read thirty-five in a day on Sunday in the office, but I don't want to spend (this) Sunday in the office. Hair falls every time I get dressed, change my shirt or undershirt, or even touch my head. More tea.

Squirrels romp and shiver at once on the ice-slick tree branches outside, where freezing rain is falling, through thick mist, on the snow.

Gambier, Ohio, February 22, 1993

6:45 A.M. Exhaustion hit me yesterday. I got into bed, fully dressed, and slept from 3 P.M. until 4:45, when I got up and called KJ while the weekend rates were still on, just under the wire, to say I'd spent Sunday with *KR* work, and my own notebooks, but I was tired, more afraid in the isolation I felt, hated my hair falling out...

—and now it's ten to seven in the evening. I came home from

the office at four, because that's when Nadine was leaving the library, to return there in an hour for a five-hour night shift. I must work my way up from what promises to be a major funk: the temperature is dropping back down to 15 degrees; the rain has turned into an ice storm; it snowed on and off all day, and is expected to snow tomorrow, on top of the ice, making the roads treacherous to impassable. I've no idea if the Columbus oncologist will be able to get to Mount Vernon tomorrow, or if, after seeing me, he'll give me my treatment. When I touch my head, more hair falls out, and in one out of every ten of the short stories and poems I read in the *KR* manuscript pile, someone dies or is dying of cancer.

I brought home manuscripts—have read twelve out of twenty or so, which depressed me more, not because of the above, but because of the general level of competent mediocrity. What a relief when there's work by a nurse, an electrician, a bus driver, whose ideas have developed through living and reading—not in creative writing workshops. (Last week there was an imperfect short story crackling with talent and energy by a telephone linewoman.)

I could take a shower, and have half of what's left of my hair come out (it will come out whether I take a shower or not). KJ's on call tonight. Iva canceled dinner this evening: she's working on the lighting for a play all week, and has a chemistry test coming up. We'll have lunch on Saturday before her Chamber Singers concert.

Besides Iva, I feel as if Nadine is the only person in Gambier who cares if I'm sick or well, coping, miserable, or moribund— and I may be wearing her down "hitchhiking" to work and back with her, tagging along on her Saturday morning supermarket runs (often the highlight of my weekend), getting lifts to the Mount Vernon pharmacy. I could call Anne Shaver in Granville— to talk to someone else in Ohio who'll (metaphorically) look me in the eye.

JS in the English department (a single woman my age, and declared feminist) has said maybe three sentences to me in three years. When I first came back, two weeks ago, she stopped (thrust her head, but not her feet) in my office to say how sorry she was, etc. She was due for a mammogram herself. "We're all just waiting for the axe to fall." Perhaps we could have lunch? I said. But I didn't suggest a date—and she's never taken me up on it.

A, B, C sent me "get well" cards in New York: everybody was told about the mastectomy—and I know it was Y who made sure of that. They say "hello" in the hall, sometimes ask how I'm feeling. But never "let's have lunch" or "come to dinner"—as if "it" were catching, as if someone "in my condition" couldn't possibly want companionship.

Y did, on her card, offer me lunch at the Pine Tree Barn.

I'd like a glass of wine I "shouldn't" have—now, not because it's fattening, but because "they say" drinking wine may provoke breast cancer. How I hate the idea that drinking wine with dinner, common as bread or morning coffee in France or Spain or Italy or Portugal, "gave me cancer"! Have three babies before you're thirty, *don't* have children after you're forty; don't eat meat, cheese, butter, eggs, or cream; don't take birth control pills: what a life proposed for women. And, of course, avoid coffee and tea and "alcohol."

Gambier, Ohio, February 23, 1993

5:30 P.M. Nadine's coming to dinner at 8—the least I can do to acknowledge her generosity, have some good company, and use the salmon steaks I took out of the freezer when I thought Iva was coming.

Dr. Ungerleider is a rotund, white-haired chap in a herringbone jacket and red tie, whom I rather liked. He asked me the usual "personal" questions, and I cited KJ by name to him (and to the nurse) as my "life partner" and told Dr. Ungerleider that she was training as a P.A. After he did all his paperwork, he turned around

from the desk on his swivel chair, and said, "About your partner..." ("Now, are we in for it?" I thought.) "Is she thinking of
moving here to join you? Would she be interested in working in
the Oncology SICU [Surgical Intensive Care Unit] in Columbus?
They want to hire two P.A.'s there." That's the James Cancer
Clinic, one of the best in the country. He gave me the name and
number of the director. KJ *could* conceivably do her SICU rotation
there, to see how she liked it. Castles in the air, counting
unhatched chickens. But it's a possibility!

Clearly I'm much more "up" than when I didn't know if I'd get
the treatment or not (I did!). I wrote to Geneviève. I began reading *KR* manuscripts I'd brought home with me. Rafael's essay on
AIDS and poetry came in today's mail. Chip called to say the *New
Yorker* turned down his Harlem/Hart Crane novella—so I'll use
two chapters in the *KR*. Nepotism be damned: we need good,
"known" fiction writers.

Gambier, Ohio, February 26, 1993

10:30 A.M.—eleven manuscripts read, cold, snow...I'm not
exactly taking a morning off, but working in the apartment.
There's a search committee meeting with the third managing editor candidate at 2: someone will pick me up at 1:30. Eat
"lunch"—a bran muffin and coffee; take Cytoxan and vitamin C
pills.

The positive side of all this: I've come to enjoy this apartment
more, to take shelter in it. I look with pleasure at the local handmade quilt wall hangings I've collected, the art gallery posters I
sent from Paris and had framed. I live in all of it: write and read
in the study/second bedroom, meditate, exercise, very occasionally entertain in the living room, sleep in the bedroom in the sec-
ondhand bargain oak bed, on crisp blue-and-russet geometric
print 200-thread sheets I chose (tossing and turning, asleep at
10:30 P.M. but wide awake at 2 A.M. and fitful for the next two and
a half hours).

Paris, July 1995

Eleanor Bender, then the Director of Development at U.C. Davis, came to Kenyon at the end of February as a development consultant for the *Kenyon Review*, funded by the Lila Wallace marketing grant. She was to spend some working hours "below decks" with me and Y, but the main purpose of her visit was to meet with the college's administrators to plan fundraising strategies for the magazine. Her visit had been planned in the fall, scheduled while I was recuperating in New York. But the college president hadn't made room for her on his calendar, and the day to be spent brainstorming with the development office shrank to a couple of hours, during which Eleanor was essentially told that the college did not believe in "targeted fundraising." Any money raised specifically for the magazine would have to come from our—that is my—own initiatives. (To my own amazement, and thanks in part to Eleanor's advice, I raised $43,000 from individuals and foundations in the next eight months!)

We were old acquaintances from Eleanor's *Open Places* days at Stephens College; she stayed with me in Gambier in my study/spare room. After years of post-divorce midwestern isolation, at fifty-two she'd remarried, to a scholar of Asian history. I'd last seen her in September, at a brainstorming conference in San Francisco for the grant, looking glowing and fit. She'd renewed her literary connections by acting as a consulting poetry editor for the *KR*.

During her stay, a memorial celebration for Audre Lorde had been arranged by the new Women's Studies director, at the (equally new) Multicultural Center, a porched white frame house on a wide lawn set back from the center of campus. It was in the early evening—very cold, but dry. (I was glad we had Eleanor's rental car). Laurie had asked me to speak about Audre as I'd known her—everyone thinks I knew her better than I did—read some of her poems, perhaps something of my own, and encourage the students also to read aloud from and discuss her work. (Laurie knew, of course, that I was being treated for the disease which finally defeated Audre: it's only now that I wonder if any of the students knew that, too.)

When we arrived, the main room—once the large living room of a Midwestern home—was crowded with students, mostly women, all white but for one Latina and one light-skinned black girl, sitting on every available sofa, chair, radiator cover, windowsill, the floor. Laurie and a cadre of Women's Studies students had provided soft drinks, crudités, cookies, coffee. No one from the English faculty came—Laurie was the only teacher present. A seminar in African American literature, taught by one of Kenyon's three black faculty members, met at that very hour—but, as he'd told me in the English office, "Richard Wright was being discussed that session."

I spoke briefly about Audre's work: her poems, her essays, her presence. I read three of her poems, and for the first time, "Year's End," the poem I wrote in November after Eleanor had called and told me of Audre's death, before my own diagnosis. I asked the students to speak. Several young women—the black student, the Latina student, and three or four others—had brought books of Audre's poetry, or *Zami*. There was mention of Audre's "universal relevance": "despite" her lesbianism, her militant Afro-Caribbean-American feminism (upon all of which she insisted in any discussion) as non-black, non-lesbian students hesitantly tried to affirm their entitlement to their own responses.

It probably would have infuriated Audre, and inspired some of her more brilliantly belligerent pedagogy. Had I been in better form, I might have been able to open a discussion of Audre's insistence on her particularities—and given some context for her work, among that of African American poets, feminist poets, poets *tout court*. But I'd used up all the energy I had.

Gambier, Ohio, March 3, 1993

I had the second cycle/second I.V. treatment yesterday. At the Mount Vernon hospital it's delivered with an I.V. needle, not a butterfly. And the oncology nurse couldn't find a vein. She tried twice, with me sitting in a chair designed for I.V. chemotherapy delivery, and thus anxiety-producing in itself, in an extremely cold room. She commented on how thick my skin was, and how small my veins. It hurt like hell each time she thrust the needle in; she left it in both times, and both times said she wasn't getting a blood return. Finally, she went out to get another nurse, leaving me in the chair, in the cold, so I would "relax." If I'd only "relax," my veins would be more prominent, and not constrict. The second nurse, a larger, also florid and middle-aged woman, knelt on the floor and drove the needle into my arm up to the plastic hilt. There was indeed a "blood return"—blood spurted out all over my hand and wrist, all over the chair arm. The vein had collapsed around the needle, she said, but at least she didn't remove it and start again: the saline solution I.V. began to drip; the first nurse shot in her two cylinders of what we hope is purifying poison. Twice she exclaimed that I'd be glad not to see *her* again, which won't help when I *do*, in April or May. I asked why it couldn't be done with a butterfly needle, as it was in New York, and was told, "That's not how we do it *here.*" I should never have pronounced the name "New York," just inquired in all innocence about butterfly needles.

Nadine had driven me to the hospital; afterwards (she'd been uneasy I'd been in there so long), I went with her to Ike's Diner, across from the shopping mall, and had lentil soup and half an English muffin. Then she took me home. I lay down from 1:30 until 4, got up, read *KR* manuscripts and then *The Nation*, feeling increasingly tired and unwell: a bad taste in my mouth, not nausea but the brink of it, like morning sickness all day long. I had a small bowl of bran flakes with my Cytoxan and Compazine and went back to bed at 7:45. And I still felt worn out at 7 A.M. I'm having a heavy period, with unaccustomed cramps—chemo-induced, as I wasn't due to menstruate again until the twelfth or thirteenth.

Ten to five, up from a nap that was, really, lying on my back with my eyes closed. As I heated water for tea, Jennifer, the student intern, came by with the English muffins—and a little pot of cheerful purple crocuses. In the afternoon I slogged on with the sonnets—with which I'm not too thrilled. Interweave them with a set built around the hospital? I'm disinclined to tell the too-familiar story of breast lump discovery and its attendant events—in sonnets. But it's better than sleeping, better than reading another thirty manuscripts, better than imagining Y's resentment hissing like steam from her office downstairs as the English department conviviality drifts through my office door.

Gambier, Ohio, March 7, 1993

Iva came to dinner on Friday night, after her choir rehearsal. I'd spent almost three hours doing laundry. It was almost seven when I got back, through the snow, so tired I couldn't imagine being hungry, even in an hour and a half. But I talked to KJ on the phone, *didn't* take a nap, and marinated pork chops in red wine, a teaspoonful of soy sauce, and mustard, made curried string beans: the thought of curry revived my appetite.

Iva was cheerful and loquacious. She'd read *Beloved* for her English course: "the best book I've ever read!" The sane and charismatic grandmother, Baby Suggs, reminded her of her own centenarian great-grandmother Boyd: that's what she'd written her essay about. What other Morrison novels could she read? I gave her $10 for *Sula* or *Song of Solomon* in paperback.

I'm gratified at her "claiming her identity"—at Kenyon, of all places. But it's more significant to her here than in multicultural New York, another significance entirely than at Bronx Science, where the political black kids were so color-oriented that Iva was told more than once that "she wasn't really black"—and neither was her father!

Meanwhile I ate a pork chop and curried beans and Iva ate nothing. I took two sips of my glass of Côtes du Rhone and poured the rest back into the bottle (which no one else would be touching). Iva got up and hugged me and said, "What's happened to my Mommy? I want my (big old loud wine-guzzling) Mommy back!"

Vitamin pills, Cytoxan, a cup of bouillon to wash it down. Marie's in Paris now, at my studio: we had a long talk yesterday that did me good. She had lunch with the Migrennes at Fandango; she's having dinner with Geneviève on Tuesday: otherwise she's sitting at the pine table working on poems, then taking long walks. There are primroses and pansies in the Vert-Galant; magnolias in the rue Charles-V.

The sun's going down: I got lost in the memory of the young woman across the street at 26, rue de Turenne, pregnant in November, pensive at her kitchen table in an oversized white T-shirt while the rotund, elderly mom-and-pop upstairs were having a raucous extended family dinner, all their windows across the street opening those lives into mine.

Paris, July 1995

I finished my six cycles of chemotherapy in late June, and returned to France for two and a half months (with the "blessing" of the new managing editor) where I completed the manuscript of *Winter Numbers*. In the fall of 1993, the trustees of Kenyon College began an "investigation" of the *Kenyon Review*. KJ graduated from the Harlem Hospital Physician Assistant program and went to work there with AIDS patients—her goal in this mid-life career change. In April 1994 it was announced that the *Kenyon Review* would continue with a reduced subsidy. In May I was informed that my own contract (up in June) would not be renewed.

The baby across the street is walking. My own health is, so far, touching my wooden worktable, good.

Mimi Schwartz

❦

The Other Redhead and Me

IN 1988, SIX WEEKS AFTER MY MASTECTOMY, I WAS feeling pretty good again. Breast cancer, I decided, was not what I thought after years of reading articles like "Victims in Terror" and "The Anguish of Women with Breast Cancer." Since my surgery, I hadn't read one. Why should I? I had lost a breast (lumpectomy was not an option in 1988 because the cancer was multi-foci, the doctor said) and I hated the scarred emptiness. But I didn't need chemotherapy; I had a husband who said, "It's like making love with two women. What's bad about that?" And I never could wear a bikini anyway.

"You stay and read," I told Stu as he eyed a table of pamphlets under a Reach for Recovery banner: "Breast Cancer: Facts & Figures," "Cancer Check-Ups," "A Call for Help." I wanted none of them. We were at a conference on breast cancer and two hundred people, mostly women over forty, were chatting like old friends around giant urns of decaf coffee. "Everyone looks so healthy!" I said, elated. There was no doom and gloom here, no hysteria, just as I suspected. The media really did hype women's hysteria much more than that of men who had heart attacks. "I'm going to talk to people. Maybe I'll write this up." I wanted the world to know how well we women coped.

Over by the display of bathing suits and prostheses, an elegant, red-headed woman in a charcoal gray pants suit was thumbing through a bathing suit rack of high-cut mastectomy designs. I started thumbing too, not that I planned to buy one. You could sew a special pocket into a normal suit, a friend had told me, and I was going to do that when I started swimming laps again. Maybe the following week. No reason not to, my doctor had said.

I smiled. "Your first conference?"

"My third," the red-headed woman said, holding up a silky blue print. I liked her hair color, auburn like mine, and that cobalt blue was good on me, too. She smiled. "I've been on chemo for three years and I'm thinking it might be too much. One of these workshops might tell me."

"Three years?" I stepped back. That's absurd.

"Yes. My doctor wants to keep me on it." Her voice sounded casual. "But I don't like the tiny blood clots under my skin. And my hair isn't growing back." She held a purple bathing suit to her chest and turned toward the mirror, tilting her head.

I saw freckles, not clots, on her hands and wrists. Was that beautiful hair really a wig? "My doctor at Columbia Presbyterian is terrific, very understanding. Maybe you need another opinion," I said. I kept pressing. "You should call him." I noticed her wedding band. "Maybe your husband could drive you." I wanted her to whip out a pen and paper and write my great advice down, but she was admiring a velour two-piece.

"My husband had a nervous breakdown. He still hasn't recovered, although he is home from the sanatorium."

"That can't be!" I said it before I could stop, and felt myself tailspin the way I did when I saw a blotch on my thigh the week before. Luckily the doctor assured me that it wasn't melanoma.

"Well, good luck!" I smiled, planning my escape. "I hope you get your answers."

"You too."

She turned back to the rack, selecting a pink print with a sarong top while I fled to the table of mini-muffins being served on huge, silvery platters. Stu was there talking to no one, smart man. I told him about the three years of chemotherapy, the nervous breakdown, the deep worry lines I did not see because I liked auburn hair, which was really a wig.

"Still, she's coping—or she'd be at home, wringing her hands like her husband." *My* husband took a poppy seed muffin the size of a very fat cherry.

"But she should be finding another doctor, not a bathing suit," I snapped.

Beside us, two trim women in tight, blue-white perms—they could be sisters—were chatting with a tall woman in a straw hat covered with paper flowers. I could not see her face but she laughed from her belly as a bran muffin disappeared under the wide brim. "Have one," Stu said, holding a bran and lemon poppy in his palm. "They're both good."

"No!" I was furious. I wanted the red-headed woman's life under control, not the pretense of a wig and a smile. I thought of my mother always prepping me to *smile:* people don't like sour faces, especially on a girl. "You'll feel better," she'd say, which would make me scowl more. The pressure of cheerfulness always got me down. I'm a dud on New Year's Eve.

The bell rang for the workshops; we headed for breast reconstruction, first ballroom on the right. The speaker was a plastic surgeon, very upbeat, who showed videos and slides about what could be done. Forty of us were scattered in a cavernous room of red velvet chairs under chandeliers glittering in celebration. The building was a wedding palace most days.

"I can have sixteen-year-old breasts again, no sag," I whispered to Stu. "If only my other one looked like that. I like symmetry." He squeezed my hand and I looked for the red-headed woman, who wasn't there.

Three seats over sat a pretty young woman not more than twenty-five, with long blond hair, definitely her own. She had on the kind of angora sweater I used to wear in sixth grade when overnight I became a 34C and wanted the boys to notice. I resisted

looking at her chest; she must be here with a mother or grandmother who was somewhere else.

Behind her, nearer to me, sat a husky, moon-faced woman with
a large mole on her cheek, my age. Now *she* looks as if she's had
cancer, I thought. She was solemn, no smile, not even a scarf to
cover the inch of gray-black bristle on her head. She had on a men's
shirt, loose, and was taking lots of notes on a yellow legal pad. She
stopped to interrupt the speaker: "Aren't these implants cancer-
producing? A new report says that—"

"I use only saline-filled molds," the doctor said quickly.
"Perfectly safe."

"Bull!" I heard behind me. I knew it was the woman with the
mole without turning around.

"How long until the scars fade?" It was a buxom woman, mid-
forties, to my left. She had on a red power suit and a red plaid turban. Nice hat.

"We have excellent luck with saline. Most women say they don't
notice them after a while."

"Even with keloids? My scar is so red." It was the pretty blond
woman. Damn, I thought. She wasn't much older than my daughter.

"We've had good luck. Believe me."

"Bull!" I heard again, louder this time. The young blond
turned around to stare and bodies shifted as cynicism made us
ugly again.

At lunch we were directed to a large round table for ten in a
room of twenty such tables. I was hoping the woman in a flowering caftan and turban—tall, noble, powerful—would sit next to
me, but I got the "Bull" woman. Across the table, a thin, high-
pitched woman was chattering about low-fat recipes which she was
gathering into a cookbook. She'd be happy to send us all one.
"George here wants me busy, right, sweetie? He won't allow me to
be sad." She looked at a small, dimple-cheeked fellow eating black
olives off the relish tray. "He says that once you let sadness start, it
keeps growing and will take you over."

She beamed and I shivered. Susan Sontag was right. It was cancer growing in that metaphor, not sadness, as if the wrong mood could do you in. And if it did it was your own damn fault, according to George and the self-help book the woman was now recommending, on and on, gaily. "Dr. Siegel saved my life, didn't he, sweetheart? It's so amazing how the mind rules the body. Cheerfulness is the secret, you know."

She giggled and I scowled, thinking how often I'd wept, looking in the mirror. And how the night before, Stu had lassoed my naked waist from behind, kissing my neck, then the tears, and whispering I smelled good.

I stared at the chef salad, the tears coming again.

"These rolls are better than they look." The woman with the mole passed me the bread basket. "Usually institution food stinks."

"No, thanks really. I'm watching it." I'd decided to look good again, at least with clothes on.

She shrugged, rearranging her yellow pad, half-covered by a napkin, on her lap. "You on chemo? That'll put the pounds on you. It did me."

"Really? I thought you lost weight with it." I had visions of wasting away even though my friend Doreen looked fine.

"Yeah, I put on twelve pounds in six months." She spread her roll with the fake butter; they had announced its purity over the loudspeaker. "But I don't care. No one else is sharing my bed lately. My lover left when I lost my hair. Dumb, right? The breast didn't seem to matter."

I touched Stu's arm, but he was engrossed in a woman in a Navy uniform on his right, and opposite me George's wife was urging everyone into Yoga therapy. "Have you been off chemo long?" I asked the mole woman dutifully. She was eating another roll, spreading fake butter with a vengeance.

"A month this time, but I gained last time, too."

"You had it twice?"

"Yeah, ten years ago, but this time the lump was benign. I did chemo just to be safe."

That sounded insane, but I was through crusading. My doctor, I told myself, knew what he was doing. I concentrated on cutting my salad. The loudspeaker went on: "Our egg-free custard is approved by the Cancer Nutrition Society. Enjoy, ladies." Stu stopped talking to the Navy woman. Interesting lady, he told me. She was going to re-enlist for another five years and then open a motel in Delray Beach with her brother-in-law. It was on the bend where that good fish restaurant was, the one with the great Caribbean chowder. The Navy woman overheard his enthusiasm and winked at us. "She just made a down payment."

"How long ago did she have cancer?" I hated asking, but it was a reflex around here.

"Six months ago, but she's like you. In good shape."

"I'll bet," I muttered.

He kept on. "She went to the workshop on chemotherapy and said the speaker was recommending it for everyone. New findings from the National Cancer Institute. She was calling her doctor tomorrow."

"Well, I'm not calling anyone," I snapped. "My doctor knows what he's doing. He's head of the program, isn't he?"

Someone put coffee and the egg-free custard in front of me. I pushed it toward Stu. "It's approved by our cancer nutritionists," the waiter said proudly. I was desperate to leave. I should have gone to my office and cleaned out two months of junk mail. "If my doctor thought I needed chemotherapy, he would have said so." I tipped the coffee cup, which flooded the saucer.

"No one said you should call him," Stu said evenly. No baiting him today.

The legal pad was now propped against the table and the woman with the mole was writing in big, sprawling letters; I tried to read it.

...The red-headed woman next to me is acting like she shouldn't be here. But who the hell should? She keeps hanging on to her husband's arm as if he could save her from all this...And she smiles a lot. Must be scared to death.

Scared and smiling, me? I'd been Joan of Arc before today, convinced that if I burned at the stake, it would be a fearless spectacle to the end. But that was when doctors knew everything, I didn't have choices, and Death wasn't sitting in every chair in this room.

"Okay, I'll call him tomorrow," I said, reaching for Stu's arm. I stopped. "I don't want you blaming me later...If only she'd done this! What was she thinking of?"

"No one is blaming you."

"Not now, but you will. Nothing bad can just happen."

The woman stopped writing and looked up. "The healthy sons of bitches need a reason, right?" She grinned.

"You a writer?" I asked, looking at her pad and thinking we could join forces. I needed some no-nonsense fury.

"This? No. I like reading it over at night. Life doesn't suck as much because everybody's got problems, right?" She stood up to go, patting my shoulder. I was surprised at how short she was. "Well, hang in there. I'm going to check out macrobiotic counseling, see what magic they offer." She laughed. "Take care."

"You too."

I expected a brisk walk, but she moved slowly with a slight limp, and I stood up quickly to go. I was through with cancer, present tense. All I wanted was the blue chair of my living room, a little Mozart, and light streaming in through the window.

On our way out, I saw the other red-headed woman in her charcoal pants suit. She was sitting next to the doctor who lectured on breast reconstruction. She was listening intently while he did the talking, and she smiled just as I pointed her out to Stu. "You're right, you'd never know. They could be on a date," he said, taking my arm as we walked through the double glass doors.

*

Dr. Smith insisted that I didn't need chemotherapy. So did one out of two second opinions, so I picked the advice I wanted to hear and guessed right. I'm here eleven years later, and now I am deciding whether to stop taking tamoxifen and start estrogen so my bones won't crumble and my heart won't collapse in ten years. My gynecologist is for it, my oncologist says don't risk it, and my surgeon, Dr. Smith, who was my old fountain of wisdom, quit treating women with breast cancer and is now working in a V.A. hospital.

The flyer for this year's New Jersey Conference on Breast Cancer is on my desk, but I won't go. I still need the aura of natural well-being and the illusion that cancer and death are distant cousins, barely related. "Look at me, I'm fine!" I assure women who find a lump and call me for advice, gathering stories so they can feel in control. I tell them about my friend who had ten malignant nodes and a year of chemotherapy three years before me. She's fine. And about my colleague who had a double mastectomy two years before that. Fine. And about my old roommate's mother who lost a breast at thirty-five and just celebrated her eighty-fifth birthday. These good stories need to be the norm, nothing unusual, just what happens to us women who cope. Then the still-red scar, the ache that lingers after a hot shower, even the sad, unlucky stories hovering behind a brave smile or an angry "Bull!" all fade into daily life, and I am a woman who just made a new recipe for cream-of-pear soup (with tofu) and is looking for a bathing suit in black velour—with a built-in prothesis pocket I won't have to sew in.

Carol Dine

Poems

Genetics

*The healthiest way of being ill is one most
purified of metaphoric thinking.*
                                    —*Susan Sontag*

In surgery,
they opened and closed
my father. Afterwards,
the doctor drew a diagram
of the intestine
where cancer had detoured—
the winding was a tunnel
with no way out.

My friend shot a snake. The arrow
went through the middle of the body
impaling it to a log.
Writhing against the shaft,
the snake split itself open.
I remember the sun
shining down on the babies.

I inherited his long legs,
the brownness of his eyes,
his Russian moods.
I imagine him as a juggler.
He throws the bastard gene to me.

I dreamt I was a snake that night.
It had a mouth at its head,
another at its tail,
and each mouth, facing inward,
was eating its own skin.

My breast is marked
for surgery. When I awake,
I will step out of this metaphor,
this discarded skin.

I've slid three times
from the knife,
each time, delivered
of a new self, lighter.

Freestanding

I have a breast that's sculpted
from the skin of my back.
If there are two pink roses
on a stem,
it's the one that's faded.

In semi-darkness, once I saw
a dancer arch the highway of her back.
The spotlight came up
like a full moon. Naked
to the waist, she faced the audience—
she had one breast,
beside it, a horizontal scar.
She raised her arms above her head
like a column, twirled; the breast
appeared, disappeared.

Circles

1.

Ash Wednesday and everywhere
there are circles
like the one on the forehead
of my lover when he parted
his blonde hair.
I called it the kiss of Jesus.
Later he was lying in the open
coffin, and I thought I saw it
reappear.

2.

When Rubens painted the eternal
dot on the breast
of a naiad,
it was as if the pigment were wet
light.
The master knew it was all illusion,
the goddess wading
pink as a Nerine lily
in her opulent flesh.

3.

Tomorrow, I will remove a bandage
unveiling
the plastic surgeon's rendering—
my tattooed nipple
that cannot be
suckled or aroused.
Then in the mirror
I will face the body
and the body's unrequited desire
for what's been given up.

❧

From the Front Line

I AM IN A SMALL BOAT FLOATING ALONG THE INSIDE of my body. My body is a river. The river is burning. The territory on the banks has been pillaged and razed. I assess the damage: sexless organs, intact—lung, liver, kidney. But there's a hollow where the breast should be. Every female part, gone—uterus, ovaries, fallopian tubes. In the shallows, I moor the boat, hear the dead calling: "You belong with us. Come."

I have had breast cancer three times. For nineteen years, I have tried to write my way through to the other side of terror. In the act of writing, I was also sustaining my body. I deliberately avoided references to cancer as war. My back went up when I read the obituaries: "She died after a lengthy battle with breast cancer." When the American Cancer Society presented me with the Sword of Hope Award for a newspaper article, I wished the rapier on the plaque were a gladiolus. Still, looking over my essays, journals, and poems about my breast cancer, I discovered that without meaning to, I have been a war correspondent—the battleground, my body.

1980. Malignancy, under two centimeters, right breast: Lumpectomy, twenty-three external beam treatments to the breast and lymph nodes; iridium implant.

This was the beginning.

Walk through the door...into the vapors, the steam. On a metal table, lie perfectly still. Underneath my knees, a pillow rolled like a

sandbag. Over my head, huge gray arm of the machine. Lights go out.
Wheels on the gurney move back and forth, back and forth. Count
one, two. Then a high-pitched sound from fifty holes aimed at my
breast. No heat, no pain. Pain would be easier than this slow shrinking of flesh.

(from "On Navigating the Shoals of Breast Cancer," *Boston Sunday Globe,* May
30, 1982)

I told it as it was, reporting with precision both the facts and my
feelings about what was happening to my body. I almost believed
that this account could contain the cancer, a reinforcement of the
radiation therapist's assurance that I was cured. When I asked him
if he were certain, he said that with these treatments there was a 95
percent chance that the cancer would not recur.

1985. Infiltrating ductal carcinoma with extensive lymphatic
small vessel invasion. Mastectomy right breast, latissimus flap
reconstruction. Chemotherapy, CMF (Cytoxan, methotrexate, 5-
fluorouracil), six months.

Escalation. Poison chemicals. Sometimes right before an injection I'd imagine the drugs in shapes of tiny boxing gloves, or vora-
cious mouths devouring the bad cells. Then I'd go to my mother's
house, to the room of my childhood, to write in my journal. I was
more than a cancer patient. I was a witness. The writing made me
face my fear of dying and at the same time distanced me, as if I
were telling the horror of someone else's body.

April 19. C (Chemo) Day. The nurse calls my name out loud. I follow her down a corridor through the sweet smell of chemicals like
perfume gone bad. The rooms are all the same. Now I'm sitting in
a chair, I'm out of my body. She flicks a vein in my left arm. This
is it. Needle, the burning. My head is light and spinning . . . .

May 13. I am losing strands of hair. I find them everywhere—on
my pink dresser tray, on the rim of the bathtub. They are scattered
on my pillow like dark spokes of a wheel. I want to count them and

put them back on my head. Instead, I gather them up one by one, hold them in my palm for a minute like a prayer.

(from "Treatments: A Journal," *Boston Sunday Herald,* April 30, 1989)

In the years following the chemo, which brought me to menopause at age forty-two, to prevent cancer from taking over my life, I wrote a book of poems called *Trying to Understand the Lunar Eclipse* (Erie Street, 1992). I needed a safe place for my art to go. My poems were about the constant in nature: the mercy of tides, hedges of beach roses, the wall of buoys at Barnegat Harbor. I wrote about learning to sail, drifting as a state of mind. I was trying to eclipse my cancer.

1993. Right proximal femur, metastatic adenocarcinoma, consistent with breast origin. Deep excisional biopsy of right hip malignancy, stabilization with bone cement and plate; radiation.

The dreaded cell was loose in my bones like a live grenade. Now I could no longer separate myself from the cancer. I was becoming the cancer. My breast, my femaleness, had placed me in severe danger. This was not safe to record in the Sunday newspaper. I could not tell my secret to the world: metastasis—my inadequacy was spreading. I wrote about it in code, in poetry. To reduce the shame, I identified with Frida Kahlo, who reveled in her body's suffering.

> They've cracked us open
> like earth, Frida,
> like a hope chest.
> The moon has risen,
> and the mottled sun.
> They've pruned us like branches
> of the Guayacan.
> Your spine has been soldered, Frida.
> There's metal in my hip.
> Both of us clang when we walk,

take turns recovering
on hospital trolleys.

(from "Arbol de la Esperanza," *Sojourner,* May 1996)

I moved in two worlds unsure of whether I belonged among the living or the dying. I began to do research on Mesoamerican burial customs. I traveled to the Yucatan, to the ruins of Chichen Itza, Tulum, and Coba, where I listened for voices. Then I began poems inspired by photographs of the mummies of Guanajuato, Mexico. I was preparing myself should I have to enter the country of the dead.

At first you cannot look at the dead:
the gravity of open mouths,
a valley rising
between a woman's breasts.
Think of the hips
as a map spread before you.
Do not be afraid.
The dead walk in their sleep,
reappear as gardens.
Think of the dead
as landscape,
as still life with bones.

(The Bitter Oleander, Spring 1999)

Poems about the army of the dead also provided an outlet for my rage which I did not dare express to God.

Some of the dead are defiant.
They stand against the living
at the barricade.
Their fists are clenched.
The arms are longbows or spears.
Their hearts are bedrock.

(from *Light and Bone/Luz y hueso*)

1995. Surgical Pathology Report: 51-year-old female with a history of breast cancer metastatic to the right hip, who now presents with post menopausal bleeding....Received fresh in the Frozen Section Lab, uterus, cervix, right ovaries and right fallopian tubes. No diagnostic abnormalities recognized.

This time, luck; no evidence of cancer. But after the hysterectomy, I felt desexed. My womanhood had been delivered between my legs. I wrote in my journal: *"I have been robbed; I tell them I will not press charges if my belongings are returned.*

"I imagine a junk yard filled with small breasts piled up like hub caps, yards of fallopian tubes, enough parts to make a whole new woman." Language could not capture the emptiness. I tried humor. *"You know the photograph of Marilyn Monroe from* The Seven Year Itch? *She's straddling the subway grate in her billowy dress; the sex goddess is smiling. Well, if I stood there beside her, the draft would travel straight on up, I'd open my mouth and whistle like an old tea kettle."*

To get myself back, I filled envelopes with poems—*do you want me*—and walked slowly to the post office. One day I no longer felt like a shadow. I moved to an apartment across from the ocean. Watching the full moon rise over the waves, feeling the undertow, I was ready to be loved.

I answered a personal ad from the newspaper. I met a stranger. He kissed my hair. I was scared to be naked. "I have breast cancer," I said. "Let me wrap my wing around you," he said. I undressed. Tongue, hands, enormous heat. We undid the metaphor.

1993-1999. *Remission., n. 1. Act of remitting or forgiving.* I have. Forgiven myself. I have survived. I am not my breast cancer. I am a poet who has breast cancer. Now I follow the voices of female saints, the language of ecstasy, suffering, and faith. Saint Agatha, Saint Rosalia, Saint Mary Magdalene. I correspond with Saint Lucy, patron saint of sufferers of eye trouble and writers. Her eyes were plucked out, then miraculously restored.

Lucy, at the site
of your eyes on the altar plate,
two cold blue stones,
I wanted to hide
what was taken—
my breast, its roseate nipple,
the way I saw myself
as dying.
Then love
flared on the walls
that had been dark
as a monastery
opened
my body
bathing
in pools of light.

Janet Sternburg

❦

The Scan Chronicles

Scan—vt. 1. *To scrutinize carefully. 1987*

WALKING IN THE WOODS TODAY, I CAME TO A channel running between two lakes. I paused, accustoming my eyes to see details; reeds in the water; pine trees, mossy boulders strewn among them. The glacier, I thought, has been active here. Then I said aloud, "Please let me stay alive."

Last year at this time I was undergoing a final chemotherapy treatment. Ahead were more days of violent nausea. I had lost most of my hair and was wearing a wig. I was still weak from the operation six months before, when I had lost a breast. I was working full time in New York City's stifling summer heat, traveling a long distance to my job on subways which, when they disgorged me, left me standing at the bottom of a flight of stairs, unsure whether I could climb to the street.

Why didn't I take a break during those months of chemo? One reason was that I needed a weekly paycheck. Another was Gloria. Our friendship had left me unwilling to exempt myself from demands that had been made on her. Gloria was part of an extended Puerto Rican family that my former husband came to know when he volunteered at a South Bronx settlement house. She wasn't one of the original family of four brothers whom we helped make it from childhood to young manhood. She was my age, a single mother living in the projects, sharp and smart about most things but unable to read or write, which shamed her most deeply when her bright young son needed help with his homework.

From the first time we met, we got along; we got a kick out of one another. When she discovered a lump in her breast, it seemed natural to me, in an almost sisterly way, to find a good doctor and see her through the stages of her illness. In retrospect, though, I was obtuse. I remember going to a pharmacy with her after her chemotherapy treatment so that she could fill a prescription for anti-nausea medication. At the subway entrance, we gave each other a high five and sang a bar of that summer's hit song, "I Will Survive." Unaware of how soon the chemicals would reach her, I let her make the long trek home by herself.

She eventually had to stop working in the handbag factory, although before she left she gave me several zippered cases with French-sounding labels that belied their South Bronx origin. She relied on welfare, Medicaid, my help, and her guts. I praised her courage, which she shrugged off. Every once in a while she went on a drinking binge. She complained only toward the very end, phoning me three or four times an hour from the hospital, begging me to ask the doctors to give her stronger pain medicine even though by then she was getting doses as high as they thought a person could tolerate.

I was a little crazy after her death. My index finger swelled and throbbed so badly that I thought I'd been bitten by something venomous. The swelling went down after several days but it still reappears at times of distress. Each time, I'm struck again by what it must have been like for her to have gone through her illness alone, with the most minimal resources.

Immediately upon recovering from my final treatment, I set about having my apartment repainted, its floors sanded and stained. Although I found the process difficult, I wanted a visible symbol of recovery, and a fresh start with the man in my life. When I first told Steve that the doctor had found a suspicious lump, he responded by coming to stay with me until I got through the biopsy. He never left. Each morning I woke to his warmth and our laughter. Now that he was about to give up his beloved Village apartment and move his belongings in with mine, I said goodbye to my favorite paint scheme and schooled myself to accommodate Steve's tastes. I wanted to do what I could to keep him there beside me, anticipating a loving and companionable life together.

In the woods today, as I looked at that scene of long-ago upheaval, I asked myself questions that have haunted me since the diagnosis. If cancer were to spread beyond where I would consider living worthwhile, how would I end my life? Or would I hold onto life no matter what?

Sometimes, under the grind of everyday difficulties—and, more acutely, under a fear of losing what I love—I stop valuing life. An old pre-cancer despair takes over, and it seems to me that it would be no large loss to have a curtain clang down (I could not, at that point in the sentence, type the word "die"). At other times, I'm surprised by an almost impersonal commitment to life as when, during a screening of a war movie, I kept uttering "stupid... stupid..." at each incident that showed we actually choose to send people to their deaths.

In their intensity, my emotions remind me of how I felt as an adolescent. One worry I don't need to have is whether my emotions will dull in my middle years. I'd be a fool to take my life for granted.

Scan 2. *To glance quickly. 1989*

"Carol," I call out, "how much will the budget go up if we do that other sequence?" Carol taps the figures into her calculator. "It goes up to mmty thousand." "Can't hear you," I shout, "wait a minute until I turn over." She is sitting at the far end of the room, legs neatly crossed, yellow pad and calculator in hand, the picture of an efficient Girl Friday while I, stretched out on a metal slab while a male attendant tells me to turn toward him, am the picture—almost—of a movie producer on a masseur's table.

What's wrong with this picture? For one, I am not under ministrating hands but under a large machine that is scanning my bones. At the end of the table is a small monitor where I can see my bones fizzing as though they were carbonated. For another, the relations are entirely different. Carol and I are old friends, at work together on a documentary film. She'd accompanied me on my last round of scans and volunteered for this one too. I was about to say no, thinking that since scans will be lifelong events for me, I'd better get used to going through them alone. Then I realized that I was enormously relieved by her offer, especially since this scan is premature, three months ahead of schedule because I've had a persistent hip pain.

I'm beginning to get used to pushing in on the swing door marked Nuclear Medicine. Prepared by my oncologist, I was less disturbed than I would have been had I encountered it without warning. Still, though, it has the effect of making me feel that my body is a testing site, an atoll used for purposes that are nominally for my protection but may also be devastating. Turning onto my stomach, with my more-or-less intact but just biopsied breast still hurting, I was able to use my abdominals to lift slightly off the table and relieve the pressure. I remember the radiology technician, too. He told me about trails he'd walked in the Adirondack Mountains; afterwards he drew a map that I kept until I cleaned out the apartment that summer.

Stretched out now beneath another electronic eye, I recall words written by film director Jean Renoir after he was forced by war to leave his beloved France. He said that one must "plunge resolutely into the hell of the new world." At the end of his autobiography, he consoled himself with an old memory of floating downstream in a boat with a boyhood friend, under trees whose leafy boughs skimmed his face. He likened filmmaking to the "caress of foliage in a boat with a friend."

I'm not happy that life has taken me to this nuclear room. But here I am nevertheless, in a world turned upside down so that it is a machine that comes low and occasionally grazes my body. A strange caress, made human by a friend who shares the boat with me.

Scan 3. *To climb; derivatives, ascend, descend, transcend. 1992*

Joan and I greet each other with huge smiles, so very pleased to see one another after six months. I begin with something that had just come to me on the #104 bus: "Together we've lost about three and a half pounds since we first met." For a moment, Joan doesn't get it, and responds as to a report on successful dieting. "No," I say, patting my flat left chest and looking significantly at hers, just as flat and far more recently.

Today she is looking beautiful. I'd been a bit nervous about seeing her, afraid that her recently shaved head (a gesture of one-upping the inevitable) would make her look mannish. On one of our coast-to-coast phone calls, she had told me about her first venture out like this, to her local Soho cafe where she's a regular. The young crew-cutted waitress who floats around in a peignoir and Doc Martens had never paid any attention to her until she showed up bald. Suddenly the waitress began treating her as though she were cool, an interesting person after all.

It's all so different from when I got sick six years ago. Body mutilation has become fashionable. A photographer at a recent symposium showed images of skin-carvings, including one of herself holding a knife to her female lover's breast. The room was packed with an admiring gathering of black leather, bright yellow hair, nose rings. I stood in the back wanting to scream, "You idiots!" A knife at a woman's breast isn't a flirtation with danger. It's an attempt to stave off death.

Joan and I order coffee. I haul a shopping bag onto the café table and begin laying out a stack of scarves, flipping through them like pages of a well-thumbed book. The top one I'd recently laundered, a soft blush pink of Egyptian cotton with an ivory border. I'd ironed it especially to show how much more attractive the rest of the scarves will eventually look, even though most of them have been in my drawer for years.

I call them The Kate Wasserman Headcovering Collection, a

fond remembrance of how, when I first learned that I had to have chemotherapy, my friends sprung into action, delivering Kate to my door. Lovely Kate who had laid her head one night on her pillow and awakened to a bed in flames, later to a badly burned head which required a series of skin grafts. A woman of style and panache, Kate had invested in a remarkable panoply of head coverings.

To Joan I now show a black and white and yellow silk scarf with the initials YSL; a purple cotton triangle rimmed with gilt coins, exotic once on Kate's wide-boned face but too much for my own gypsyish features. From India, a handblocked print, burnt orange entwined with magenta, and a wrinkly turquoise scarf dotted with tiny mirrors. Next, a navy and white striped cotton square, quite smart, quite French, Jean Seberg crossed with Catherine Deneuve. A long scarf, rust-colored, with a Native American arrow motif.

I should have returned these scarves to Kate, now thriving in marriage, motherhood, and good work. But instead, I'm passing them on to Joan who, beautiful though she looks, is quite ill, at least if one judges by the number of affected lymph nodes. Hers were double mine. She's receiving chemotherapy through a drip catheter installed under her collarbone, less vein-scarring than when I received it through my hand once a month. Pulling down the collar of her blouse, Joan shows me the incision. I wince: it looks like it hurts, and it does.

Joan and I reach a point in our conversation when the thing to do is disappear into the ladies room and show each other our scars, which are more or less the same, allowing for her still-inflamed redness and the slightly more hollow dent of mine. I show her my ravishing new bra of which I am so proud, with its black lace that lets both the real and the prosthetic breast peep through. With the prosthesis slipped into its pocket like a visiting card into a glove, no one would guess I'm faking it.

It's time to leave, I'm going uptown to a show at the Guggenheim Museum. We stand outside the plate-glass window of the café, and I find myself reaching over to pat Joan's cheek, a gesture that reminds me of something my grandmother might have done. Then I'm seized with love.

In the great spiral hall of the museum, I stand for a long time looking at a piece by the contemporary German artist, Rebecca Horn. She has strung a wire from ceiling to floor. Along its length, a beat-up brown suitcase travels, ascending and descending while it slowly opens and shuts. Prayer, so often evoked in her work through that gesture of slowly coming together, again and again, like palms needing to touch.

Scan 4. *To examine minutely. 1994*

A white-coated technician picks up my chart from the reception desk and leads me down a corridor.

"Have a seat. I'm mixing up your dose right now."

She pops back in a few minutes later to tell me it will take a little longer. I ask her about the process, curious because yesterday the office had called to confirm my appointment, leaving a message saying, "If you can't come, we'll have to charge you for the isotopes we've ordered."

"Is there something active, the isotopes perhaps?"

"Yes, we get a basic kit for the test, but then we have to get the radioactive material that day from the pharmacy. We 'tag' the radioactive material to the non-radioactive—'tag' is our word for mixing—and wait until all the chemical processes take place."

She leaves. I'm waiting in a room that's buzzing loudly. The machines that surround me—consoles, screens, cameras—emit together, monophonically, like cicadas. So many scans. So many attempts to get into my veins, still collapsed from chemotherapy eight years ago. So many butterfly needles, delicate enough to succeed where blunter instruments fail.

She returns. It turns out she can't get into my veins. She keeps poking around while I read aloud. This is a technique I developed years ago, during chemo when my blood was being monitored often. I like the sound of my own voice soothing me.

This technician isn't up to the challenge my veins present and calls in the doctor. He wants to go in through my hand. We make a deal: one try and if it's too hard, we'll wait for another day. Even as I say it, I know the deal's off; he'll poke around so they can use those damn isotopes. I'm reading from a book of poetry fashioned from the diaries of pioneer women. I don't think it's the best choice; I find myself reading about a woman skinning a snake. My reading voice rises to almost a scream as he hits a bad spot. Aargh. It's over. He withdraws the needle, then himself. The technician gives me some confidential advice: "If they ever want to try the inner wrist, don't let them do it. It's the most sensitive place in the body."

These odd and lovely two hours between getting the injection and returning for the scan. Hours when the radioactive fluid is coursing through my body. When I stop to think about it, I feel like a pinball machine. Any second the silver ball of an isotope could connect with a lever and BAM! I'll light up.

I've come to enjoy these two-hour rambles. The first three or four times I was so nervous that I needed company to distract me. These days I head off alone, stopping today at a bookstore where the owner and I recommend new murder mysteries to one another. I have lunch at a Westwood café, drinking the prescribed six glasses of water and writing in my notebook about how I've asked questions of medical technicians ever since the onset of breast cancer. Knowledge has always given me a sense of control over circumstances, even when that control is illusory. But it's more than that. It really interests me to learn that an MRI can see a body in three dimensions, taking pictures slice by slice which then get assembled, like writing, into a whole story. I ask questions too because I need a scan to be more than a mechanical eye seeing inside me without any personal connection. I want to be scanned by another human being.

I get back to the office ten minutes late, and they've already taken someone else; can I come back in two hours? Since I have those radioactive isotopes racing around in my body, it seems to me that I'd just better come back, hadn't I? And I'm not going through that butterfly maneuver for a second time. I kill time. So much for enjoying time out of time. Now it's dead weight.

Finally it's my turn to go back to the room with the Nuclear Medicine sign on the door. I ask the technician if I'm going to be able to see the screen, remembering a previous scan when I'd watched, fascinated, as my bones turned into electric green fizz. She points up to a tiny TV monitor, regrettably behind my head.

"Look," she says, "just put your hand on the table." I do, but see only a dim image on the screen. I go to get my glasses from my bag and when I return, she says, "Sit down, right there." I do and look up. Sure enough, there's a big fizz on the screen. "That's your butt," she tells me.

"Is the fizz the radioactive material surrounding my bones?" I ask as I imagine isotopes zipping around my skeleton creating an outline, like a drop shadow.

"No," she says, "it's the material *in* your bones." She tells me that the camera, which now has rotated under the bed, is "attracted" to me. "If I were to sit there without the isotopes," she says, "it wouldn't be attracted to me and nothing would show up on the screen." The camera is attracted to me. Strange. I'm not attracted to it, am I?

I lie down and she straps my arms to my sides, wrapping them in a Velcro belt so that they'll stay in position. My feet are taped together. I feel as though I'm a candidate for bondage. The only thing to do is doze. Every once in a while I look up and catch the big accordion-pleated monster that houses the camera advancing toward me, stretching out its long neck like the caterpillar ride in the amusement park of my childhood. Sometimes I open my eyes and catch it minutely retracting as the camera sweeps down my anterior view, then, with a huge arcing movement, it inscribes a half circle and comes to a stop under me. It's restful, although the room's icy. She clicks off the machine and goes off, leaving me tied up.

When she returns, she's matter-of-fact, perhaps a touch disconsolate. "The camera ate your film. We have to do it over again."

"What?!"

"Yup, I took the cassette down to the processor and it ate your film. I thought it was my cassette." (Has my skeleton been reduced to the equivalent of a tape I'd rent at a video store and then find I'm playing on a faulty VCR? Yes, the answer is yes.) "I'll have to image you again."

This time it seems to take forever. I lie there imagining myself breaking the bonds and leaping from the table like a modest Superwoman. Again she trots off with the cassette and I manage to undo the constraints. I assemble myself (watch, earrings, rings), scoot to the dressing room (underpants, bra with pocket for prosthesis, sweater, slacks) and return, ready and waiting to be officially released.

She comes back, this time with that same doctor. They're carrying large-sized negatives, which they hold up against a ceiling fluorescent light in order to show me that while my posterior is fine, my anterior has clouded over. They have to do it again.

I think of bolting, never to return—anywhere—ever again! The camera, far from being attracted to me, hates me.

But I'm a good girl, a sensible one. I make a phone call to my husband telling him that I'll have to be late for the concert and return to watch the great god caterpillar make its way down my body one more time. Finally, the technician releases me, goes to check, and triumphantly brings back a set of successful images. She clips them to a lightbox and there is my skeleton; my too-narrow shoulders, my nicely balanced pelvic girdle and reassuringly symmetrical limbs. I'm strangely organless; I inquire about a few dark blobs, which she tells me are my kidneys, where I imagine the isotopes holed up, a little more time left in their half-lives. My head looks enormous. "Isn't it awfully big?" I ask. "No," she replies, "that's the way everybody is."

Scan 5. *To perceive, discern. 1996*

In the visitors' bathroom on the second floor of the hospital, I see, in the stall next to mine, in that little opening between floor and divider, a foot.

This foot is so profoundly delicate in the way that it dangles, in its espadrille (is it a shoe or a slipper... I can't tell yet) that it breaks my heart. The toe barely grazes the floor. The person is sitting on the toilet seat, but there is nothing—no force, no strength—that allows her to plant her foot on the floor, firmly, as though she were making a claim on the earth.

Instead, this foot is not exactly dangling but rather alighted as though its owner belongs neither to earth nor air, life nor death.

In the vestibule to the ladies' room, I'd seen a waiting wheelchair. Across from the stalls, a long-legged young woman in topsiders, ankles crossed, is leaning against a sink, working at carrying on a "normal life" conversation with the person next to me. "I told Glenn to go ahead with the shingling. I gave him two thousand to get started."

The voice beside me murmurs... moans... an assent? A voice so lightly tethered to conversation that at any second a windy word might lift it away.

I hear her come out of the stall, and I follow. Even though I'd known I was in the presence of someone very ill, I am shocked. Completely bald except for a little downy ducktail at the back of her neck, a young face that in healthier times must have belonged to a pretty young woman in her twenties. About her, an air of such profound sickness, such hovering...

Later, I see her in a wheelchair by the elevator, her head resting lightly on an upturned palm, eyes downcast as though death were a closer presence than her tall mustached husband standing behind her. We wait for the elevator together. I incline my head to her.

"Chemo?" I ask.

She nods, from a very great distance.

I touch my hair. "I had it too, ten years ago. I thought you'd like to know that it does pass."

She smiles a wan, unspoken thank you, an acknowledgement of a gesture sent from an asteroid, recognizable but so far away that its meaning can't matter. I blink, to hold my tears inside.

Scan 6. *To look at searchingly.* 1998

Chicken. Goose. Calf. Me. I don't even know where the liver is. Near the stomach, perhaps?

Phone call #1, four days ago. "Your blood test showed elevated liver levels, still within normal range, it's probably just the test itself, it happens all the time, the doctor wants to make sure, so can you come in for another blood test?"

Phone call #2, two days ago. "Actually it's um, more elevated, out of the normal range, it could be the result of medication you're taking, that's very common with liver elevations, can you come in as soon as possible for an ultrasound test?"

The technician, her shiny black hair curving like parentheses around her face, wants to know why I'm inquiring about the liver's whereabouts, as though she has pledged to keep even the most basic facts from the patient. For twelve years, I've been lucky; technicians have obliged. I think they find my interest flattering. The people who deal with the big machines must be solitary types, a little like writers, willing to exchange sociability for quiet darkness, for dials and screens and computers and cold rooms and turning lights on as they go into a control booth.

As she bends intently toward the shifting pixillating gray scale screen, I debate telling her that when I learned I had cancer, I became a kind of researcher. Each time I took a test, I asked question after question: "Can I look?" "Is that my collar bone?" "What's the difference between an MRI and a CT scan?" For years, I've kept a file labeled *Scanning;* a report on the latest brain scan that reveals where fake memories show themselves, a skin scanner used for detecting hidden objects. I also keep a collection of pamphlets in glossy colors, green, pink, lilac: *How Does Nuclear Medicine Work?* and *A Patient's Guide to Magnetic Resonance Imaging.* The whole culture's scanning, skimming, disclosing, and here the technician, profile close to the screen, swings the other half of her parenthesis to face me: "Why do you want to know?" She has spread colorless jelly over my diaphragm and now she's probing my ribs. "Because," I answer her, "I'm alive, so I'm interested."

It turns out that the liver is under my ribs, which are sensitive to her joystick's sliding and poking. "Turn a quarter turn to your left, please, I'm trying to get a better view of your kidney. It's clouded; did you drink milk last night?" Well, yes, not knowing it would turn to gas. She's not good at telling me when to hold my breath and when to exhale; "Breathe" is her command for everything.

We work it out. I like to show off: how chipper I am, how I make her work easier by my intelligent compliance. I hope she'll say, as others have, "You're a pleasure to work on. I only wish my other patients did as well." I'm just distracting myself with this bid for admiration, but I forgive myself, it's understandable, and she too seems to have arrived at easing up. "The liver is divided into three sections . . . now I'm looking at the left one, and I'm also getting the aorta."

She leaves the room to develop the images, first giving me a towel to wipe off the jelly. I like to do this. It makes me feel like I'm a little girl being dried off after a bath, and also like the adult who is doing the drying off.

It will take about ten minutes before I find anything out. Since my second bout with cancer, I've become acutely aware of time. I once stood in the kitchen warming something in a microwave oven and watching the timer count down from 00:30. As END blinked, I knew that those seconds will not ever be returned to me. Today as I wait through another countdown, I know once and for all: I want this life, whatever the seconds bring.

The doctor comes in. "How are you?" I ask him. "Better," he replies. He is long-faced, bearded, a familiar Jew. "Were you sick?" "No, but everyone has bad days." He bends over the dials, looking, stopping, reading, scrolling, this scholar of my own faith and my own doubts. "It's okay. I don't see a thing. You're fine." I can feel my face light up, a lovely sensation that begins in my eyes. Then his face lights up too.

Liver, liver, I'm alive. You stay there, doing your job flushing out toxins, keeping me metabolized, helping uncertainty dissolve or better yet, nourish me.

I run to the bank of pay phones to call Steve, that wonderful "good news" call. As I leave the examining room, I take one last look back; my name is on the screen above a cone swirling in shades of gray. A screensaver, perhaps, or a new technique for making a flat image appear round? Questions for another time.

Elaine Greene

❧

Telling

AT LEAST THREE TIMES IN MY LIFE I HAVE STOOD
naked in front of a mirror and squashed one breast out of the way
to see whether I could stand to lose it. Every woman must do this.

I decided I could not stand to. Every woman must decide this.

Eight days before Christmas, 8:30 A.M., I go for a routine mammogram, but after the films are developed the technician comes
back into the examining room instead of the smiling, frizzy-haired
radiologist I expect. "The doctor wants a closer look at one area,"
she says.

Uh-oh. I once heard "uh-oh" defined as the word you do not
want to hear when your doctor holds up your x-ray. Did my doctor say uh-oh? Probably not, she's too earnest. I am the clown saying uh-oh.

The area in question is on the right (the breast I always flattened
in front of the mirror) and my first thought I recognize as very odd
in view of the mortal danger I may face: It's better that it's the right
side because when my husband and I go to sleep, he curls around
me and holds me on the left.

Finally the radiologist appears, someone I have known for fifteen years. She wants to set up a needle biopsy later in the week
when the pathologist comes to the office, but I want the truth now.
Is she going to put me off so she doesn't have to deal with a bad
reaction? "Please tell me what you see," I say. Our eyes meet. I pass
the test. "Probably cancer," she says. "Percentage chance?" I ask.

"High." This is a great favor, for which I thank her—I don't need to waste any energy on a roller coaster of hope against hope. When I mention in parting that I never expected to have this disease, she smiles enigmatically and I realize everybody feels this way.

Amazingly, as though I have rehearsed all my life, an entire behavior code drops into place. I am going to be a woman of valor, I am going to be one tough lady.

Later I read the following in Anatole Broyard's book about his cancer, *Intoxicated by My Illness:* "It seems to me that every seriously ill person needs to develop a style for his illness. I think that only by insisting on your style can you keep from falling out of love with yourself as the illness attempts to diminish or disfigure you. Sometimes your vanity is the only thing that's keeping you alive." Anatole was my writing teacher and friend. We seem to have arrived independently at the same conclusion.

I will handle this my way. To begin with, nobody will know unless I tell them, and the list will be short—immediate family. People gossip about three things: sex, money, and sickness. I discover that I am passionate not to be gossiped about. I can hear the phone calls: "Oh, did you hear? Isn't it awful? I'm so upset." Upset maybe, but also excited, and can't wait to spread the news. Sicknesss is narrative, it's drama—I'm a little excited by it myself.

A note on my office door says "Doctor's appointment," and when I finally get to work, a dear and nosy colleague asks which one I went to. "Oh, the guy about my trick knee," I say.

I shut myself in my office to call my sister. Although I have resolved not to cry, not one tear, my voice box seems to be in spasm and I sound as though I am strangling. She offers to come with me for the biopsy. I accept gladly. I don't want to be seen in the waiting room with a husband. When you see a couple in a medical setting you know there is big trouble. I always look at them and write their scenarios, but sisters are not noticed.

My husband's mother died of breast cancer when he was thirteen, and his stepmother died of it twenty years later. I don't say anything about my problem until after dinner, when I invite him to sit on the sofa with me. "I have to tell you something," I say, taking his hand. My pulse must be 180. I see that my seriousness worries him; I am seldom serious. "I had a bad mammogram today and I'll have to do something about it."

"I'm so sorry," he says, looking at me hard—but calmly. After forty years of marriage, he knows how much I rely on his calmness. My brother-in-law would have his head in the oven by now. "This disease is not going to be my vocation," I say, "so give me a kiss and let's do the dishes."

That night I sleep. My sister doesn't. I think she feels it would be disloyal to sleep. After the clever pathologist manages to scoop out a few cancer cells and I still won't bat an eye, my sister uses the word "wonderful" about me. I protest that wonderful in this case merely means the patient is not standing in Macy's window screaming.

My husband and I want the children to hear the news in person. A few days later we are sitting over coffee with our elder son and his wife in their beautiful dining room. "Daddy has something to say to you," is all I can get out of my closed throat. He tells them. I haven't had my busy son's full attention like this in years. Such a solemn face. I collect some hugs and that one's over with.

Soon after, our younger son and his family are visiting us in the country for Christmas vacation. I know this tender-hearted boy will be upset so I dither about when we should drop it on them. I choose Christmas night after the children are in bed. I seat us facing each other in front of the fire, close enough to touch fingertips. I say, "And now I am going to ruin your holiday," and the voice goes, so Daddy has to do it again.

I assure both sons and their wives that I want to live and I will do whatever I have to do, and my support group is in place.

Eventful days follow during which I congratulate myself on socializing and working and having a house guest without revealing anything. There is the visit to my trusted internist. There is the visit to the surgeon my internist chooses for me, a small man with small hands whose reputation for surgery is excellent and for human relations is dismal. (Who cares? Not a woman of valor.) There is the surgical biopsy where I lose a piece of me the size of a marshmallow. There is the subsequent pathology report that includes the word "invasive." Uh-oh, I think again, as I read the page the surgeon hands me. More bad news.

This is the worst part. The surgeon will not tell me what to do. I can choose the gracelessly named lumpectomy, in which they remove more tissue at the tumor site along with lymph nodes, followed by radiation and looking down at myself and wondering for the next five years. Or, dear God, the other. It is up to me, with no medical education. I know this has to do with lawsuits. "I didn't bring my lawyer here, so why don't you send yours away," I want to say, but dare not to someone who holds a knife on me. My husband, who by now accompanies me to these consultations, can't get the surgeon to budge. I wonder why it is not considered malpractice for a doctor to refuse to share his wisdom.

My internist, despite his resemblance to Santa Claus, is a survivor of four years at Auschwitz, and he doesn't think like a lawyer. He says I have to give up the breast but that there are wonderful new reconstruction techniques. I explain to him that I don't fear dying as much as I fear waking up with *nothing there.* He says I don't have to, and sends me off to a plastic surgeon who works regularly with my breast surgeon.

The plastic surgeon is tall and handsome, expensively dressed, and known to be kind. He proposes to replace my poor ailing breast with a wedge of tissue from my abdomen and shows me one picture—of his greatest success, I presume—in which you can't tell the original breast from his creation. It's a weird scene. I am standing and wearing only an open gown and pantyhose rolled down like a bikini. He grabs a handful of skin and fat and muscle beside my navel and says, "Fine—that's enough." I am thin and have my doubts but do not voice them. He tells me the risks—

blood loss possibly necessitating transfusions, a hard recovery. I do not listen to the risks.

When I ask a question about the procedure, he shows me where the breast surgeon will cut. We are as matter-of-fact as a tailor and his customer. I lived through it, and I still think about it now and then, but I cannot say how I was able to look down as his finger traced the long path of the scalpel—right along the upper curve of a strapless prom dress—and not faint or vomit.

I have ten more days of being whole. Ten days in which to stuff myself like a Christmas goose for the plastic surgeon's raw material. It's hard work because anxiety has taken away my appetite, but I appreciate how amusing it is, the need to fatten. Says Anatole, "Illness is not all tragedy. Much of it is funny."

The office must be informed and, mindful of my unreliable voice box, I do most of it in writing—separate notes tailored to each person, but all of them say I have to be away for six weeks to undergo (unspecified) abdominal surgery. It's only half a lie, and will keep everyone's eyes off my chest when I come back.

Only once does a crack appear in the facade. On the way to a bone scan I have a friendly Haitian taxi driver named Bonhomme. I say that I like his name. We are chatting and suddenly I blurt out, "I'm very sick." He waits until a red light, then turns around to me and says, "I will pray for you." This makes me unbelievably happy.

The night before the surgery my husband stays in the hospital as long as they let him. We make easy conversation. We laugh at hospital absurdities such as making me undress and get into bed although I feel perfectly well. We eavesdrop and roll our eyes at the son patronizing his mother behind the curtain. My husband helps me keep my cool. I am grateful that he offers no special good-bye touch or glance at the breast he will not see again.

When he has to go, he says he admires me tremendously and wishes me good luck—his only wrong move. I guess I never told him how much I dislike being wished good luck, because it reminds me there is also bad luck. I never say those words to people in trouble—I say, "I'll be thinking of you" or "Blessings" or, if I know it won't be misunderstood, I make a little sign of the cross on the person's brow, something I saw Audrey Hepburn do in a movie about nuns.

An aide comes to shave one armpit and I suppress any thoughts about why this has to be done. When I go for a late-night walk through the empty corridors with my Sony Walkman playing a Louis Armstrong tape, I feel high, on the brink of an adventure. I know this is crazy and hope no nurse notices. Eventually I go to sleep.

At dawn an injection knocks me out and the adventure begins. By 2 P.M. I am back in my room feeling as though a train hit me. My husband is there and he gives me information that seems to make him deliriously happy—a daughter-in-law has learned this morning that she is pregnant. I hate his smiling face. Doesn't he see how I feel? How can he think I give a damn about anybody else? All I want is more morphine.

For three days I have private duty nurses who change my position, walk me, wash me, feed me. I need their help because four hours of anesthesia have stolen my strength, and my belly is in smithereens; the breast pain is nothing by comparison. In fact the new breast is a source of pleasure. In order to check that its blood circulation is working and the tissue is still vital, someone comes every fifteen minutes, day and night, to check the warmth of the skin. They do this by placing the backs of two or three fingers against it. It is a sweet experience—like Audrey Hepburn signing the tiny cross—one I look forward to. I can still make myself feel like a wounded creature being tenderly cared for by placing my fingers that way in that place.

The breast surgeon calls to tell me that my lymph nodes are all negative. I have been too uncomfortable to give this matter any thought but it is tremendously good news and I finally allow myself a long, convulsive crying jag, one I have to execute quietly because my roommate has three positive nodes.

The plastic surgeon and his entourage are fairly human, but I don't think I can get through to the breast surgeon. I don't even try except by being heroic. Anatole says, "If a patient expects a doctor to be interested in him, he ought to try to be interesting. When he shows nothing but . . . the coarser forms of anxiety, it's only natural for the doctor to feel an aversion. . . . I never act sick. A puling person is not appealing." Exactly. Then one morning the breast surgeon picks up a tape lying on my bed—Cecile Licad playing Schumann's *Papillons*. He says he has the Barenboim version, and we have something to talk about. Later, on my first post-operative visit, I will give the tape to him. He will promise to play it while operating. I wonder what he played for me and whether I in any way heard it.

It is frightening to leave the hospital after eight days—I have to give up being a pampered baby. But by the end of six weeks I am interested in food again. I can walk without stabbing pain, can fasten a belt around my waist without the skin feeling sandpapered. After much physical therapy I can raise my right arm to hail a cab. I can work full time, and although people may have speculated, no one told my secret. I can even wear a sweater; only a person with a morbid interest and an educated eye would detect the asymmetry, the hollow near the armpit. I don't think the plastic surgeon would show my picture to frantic new patients, though—I wasn't as fat as he thought.

I worry a little about my character when I start giving mental mastectomies to strange women in the street. Those with small, beautiful, visible breasts walking toward me get two long slashes—I know where they go. Fortunately this stops in a few weeks.

I don't let my mind wander into the realm of the actual operation until the oncologist reads to me from the pathology report: They found no other lesions. (Later my gynecologist will say when she learns this, "So you could have gotten away with it," something I had already figured out for myself.) I see that the words "fresh breast" appear on the cover page of the report. I have never seen a grislier word than *fresh* in this context and I am forced to picture the transportation of the breast to the pathology lab.

Did they put it in a plastic box? A Baggie? Did they put it on a plate, like Saint Agatha's in Italian martyr paintings? Was it still pert and round like Saint Agatha's? Not likely. Did anyone say, "Isn't this a shame, such a pretty pink nipple"? And how exactly did they determine there were no more lesions? They sliced me like a side of smoked salmon is how. Don't think sliced *me*, I say to myself. It wasn't me any more. Body parts do not have a soul.

My internist says, at my first post-operative visit, "I am in awe of your courage and equanimity." I memorize his words so I can tell my children who their mother is, but even after seven years the occasion never seems to arise.

I would have made sure to tell Anatole though, if he had lived.

Biographical Notes on the Authors

KAY BOYLE (1902-1992) was one of the last survivors of the so-called Lost Generation of expatriate writers and artists who gathered in Paris in the 1920s. She wrote more than forty books, including fourteen novels, eleven collections of short fiction, and eight volumes of poetry, in addition to essay collections, children's books, translations, ghostwritten books, and her memoirs of the Twenties. Her work appeared in magazines ranging from *This Quarter* and *transition* to *The Saturday Evening Post*, *The New Yorker*, and *The Nation*. Her honors include O. Henry Awards for Best Short Story of the Year in 1935 and 1941, two Guggenheim Fellowships, a Senior Fellowship from the National Endowment for the Arts in 1981 for her "extraordinary contribution to contemporary American literature over a lifetime of creative work," and membership in the American Academy of Arts and Letters. She was also the mother of six children and two stepchildren, and in her last three decades she was well known as a Bay Area teacher and activist.

LUCILLE CLIFTON is Distinguished Professor of Humanities at St. Mary's College of Maryland. She has received many fellowships, awards, and distinctions for her poetry collections and children's books including the Shelley Memorial Prize, the Charity Randall Citation, and an Emmy Award from the American Academy of Television Arts and Sciences. She is the only author to have two books of poetry chosen as finalists for the Pulitzer Prize in one year.

CAROL DINE has published two books of poems, *Trying to Understand the Lunar Eclipse* and *Naming the Sky*. Her work appears in *Puerto del Sol*, *Prairie Schooner*, *Women's Review of Books*, *Sojourner*, *Spoon River Poetry Review*, *Boston Globe*, *Boston Herald*, and elsewhere. For "Treatments: A Journal" she received the Sword of Hope Award from the American Cancer Society. Her bilingual manuscript *Light and Bone/Luz y hueso*, based on photographs of the mummies of Guanajuato, Mexico, was presented in a multimedia performance piece by choreographer Paula Josa-Jones at the Boston Conservatory Theatre. Carol Dine teaches at Suffolk University, Boston.

ELAINE GREENE is Features Editor of *House Beautiful*, where she edits a monthly memoir column called "Thoughts of Home." She was a design reporter for more than two decades but in recent years has become a writer of personal essays. With her husband, Lawrence Weisburg, a textbook editor, she lives in Manhattan and eastern Long Island.

MARILYN HACKER is the author of nine books, including *Presentation Piece,* which received the National Book Award in 1975; *Winter Numbers,* which received a Lambda Literary Award and the Lenore Marshall Award of *The Nation* magazine and the Academy of American Poets, both in 1995; and the verse novel, *Love, Death and the Changing of the Seasons.* Her *Selected Poems* was awarded the Poets' Prize in 1996. Her most recent book is *Squares and Courtyards.* From 1990 through 1994, she was editor of the *Kenyon Review.* She lives in New York and Paris.

JUDITH HALL is the poetry editor of the *Antioch Review.* Her first book, *To Put The Mouth To* (1992), was selected for the National Poetry Series. Her second, *Anatomy, Errata* (1998), won the Ohio State University Press/*The Journal* Award in Poetry.

SAFIYA HENDERSON-HOLMES, Associate Professor in the Creative Writing program of Syracuse University, is a poet and fiction writer. Her books are *Daily Bread* and *Madness and a Bit of Hope,* winner of William Carlos Williams Award from the Poetry Society of America. Her poetry and fiction have been widely anthologized, most recently in *Breaking Ice* and a collection of contemporary African American fiction, *Streetlights.* She happily dedicates her appearance in this book to her family.

ANNETTE WILLIAMS JAFFEE is the author of three novels, *Adult Education, Recent History,* and *The Dangerous Age.* She lives on the Delaware River in Bucks County, Pennsylvania.

MAXINE KUMIN lives on a farm in New Hampshire. She has published twelve volumes of poetry as well as novels, short stories, and essays on country living, most recently *Women, Animals, and Vegetables.* She was awarded the Pulitzer Prize for Poetry in 1973, was poetry consultant for the Library of Congress, named Poet Laureate of New Hampshire, and received the Poet's Prize in 1993, the Aiken/Taylor Award for Modern Poetry in 1995, and the Ruth Lilly Poetry Prize in 1999.

AMY LING is Professor of English and Asian American Studies at the University of Wisconsin-Madison. Poet, critic, artist, and editor, she is the author of *Between Worlds: Women Writers of Chinese Ancestry; Chinamerican Reflections,* a chapbook of poems and paintings; as well as forty-two essays published in books and journals, and poems widely anthologized. She is co-editor of seven books including *The Oxford Companion to Women's Writing in the U.S.* (with Cathy Davidson, Linda Wagner-Martin, and others), *Imagining America: Stories from the Promised Land* (with Wesley Brown), the *Heath Anthology of American Literature* (with Paul Lauter and others), and most recently editor of *Yellow Light: The Flowering of Asian American Arts.* In

1998, she was a Resident Fellow at the Rockefeller Study and Conference Center at the Villa Serbelloni in Bellagio Center, Italy.

SUSAN LOVE, teacher, surgeon, researcher, and activist, is co-author with Karen Lindsey of *Dr. Susan Love's Breast Book*, called "the bible for breast care" by the *New York Times*, and *Dr. Susan Love's Hormone Book*. She is adjunct associate professor of clinical surgery at UCLA and director of the Santa Barbara Breast Cancer Institute. As a member of the Medical Advisory Committee of the Women's Health Initiative, she helped to guide the largest study on postmenopausal women in this country.

CLAUDIA MonPERE McISAAC'S poetry and fiction appear in *Prairie Schooner, Calyx, Fourteen Hills, The Georgetown Review, The Berkeley Poetry Review, The Centennial Review,* and elsewhere. She received the 1997 *Georgetown Review* Fiction Prize, and her articles on communication appear in scholarly journals. She teaches writing at Santa Clara University and is at work on a collection of short stories set in the San Joaquin Valley.

CAROLE SIMMONS OLES has published five books of poems, including *Night Watches: Inventions on the Life of Maria Mitchell*. Her work appears in literary magazines including *Poetry, Prairie Schooner, The Georgia Review,* and *American Poetry Review*. She has received a National Endowment for the Arts grant in poetry, the Virginia Poetry Prize, and the Strousse Award. She teaches poetry at California State University, Chico, and the Bread Loaf School of English at Middlebury College.

ALICIA OSTRIKER is a prize-winning poet and critic. Her ninth book of poetry, *The Little Space: Poems Selected and New,* was a National Book Award Finalist in 1998. She is also author of *The Nakedness of the Fathers: Biblical Visions and Revisions* and *Feminist Revision and the Bible,* as well as the watershed study *Stealing the Language: The Emergence of Women's Poetry in America*. Ostriker has received fellowships from the National Endowment for the Arts, the Guggenheim Foundation, the Rockefeller Foundation, and the New Jersey Arts Council, and has won the William Carlos Williams Award of the Poetry Society of America and the San Francisco State Poetry Center Award. Her book *The Crack in Everything* was a National Book Award finalist in 1996. She teaches literature and creative writing at Rutgers University.

PAMELA POST, a fiction writer, has an MED in Psychology from Tufts and an MFA degree in writing from Vermont College. She has been teaching writing at the Fenn School in Concord, Massachusetts, for eleven years and is leading writing and healing workshops for cancer patients in the Boston area.

HILDA RAZ is editor-in-chief of the venerable literary journal *Prairie Schooner* and Professor of English at the University of Nebraska. Her most recent books are *Divine Honors,* poetry, and *Cancer in the Voices of Ten Women.*

MIMI SCHWARTZ is Professor of Writing at Richard Stockton College of New Jersey. Her books are *Writing for Many Roles* and *Writer's Craft, Teacher's Art,* as well as several regional anthologies by children, teenagers, and college writers. Her academic essays have appeared in *College English, College Composition and Communication,* and *English Journal,* and her creative nonfiction has been published in the *New York Times,* the *Philadelphia Inquirer Magazine, Lear's, Creative Nonfiction,* and *Puerto del Sol,* among others. She is currently working on a memoir/history entitled *Good People, Bad Times: Stories of My Father's German Village.*

EVE KOSOFSKY SEDGWICK is Distinguished Professor at the City University of New York Graduate Center. Her books include *Epistemology of the Closet, Tendencies, Fat Art, Thin Art* (poetry), and *A Dialogue on Love* which deals further with the experience of matastatic cancer. Sedgwick also writes a bimonthly advice column for women with cancer in *MAMM* magazine.

SANDRA SPANIER is Associate Professor of English at The Pennsylvania State University. She is the author of *Kay Boyle: Artist and Activist,* and she edited and introduced *Life Being the Best and Other Stories* by Kay Boyle and *Love Goes to Press: A Comedy in Three Acts* by Martha Gellhorn and Virginia Cowles. Currently she is editing a collection of Kay Boyle's letters, a project supported in part by a fellowship from the National Endowment for the Humanities.

JANET STERNBURG'S books include *The Writer on Her Work, Volume 1* (1981) and *Volume 2* (1991), selected for *500 Great Books by Women.* Her poems, stories, and essays have appeared in numerous journals and anthologies, most recently in *Culturefront, Common Knowledge, Screening the Past,* and *The Prairie Schooner Anthology of Contemporary Jewish Writing.* Her work in film and theater includes producing and directing a public television film on Virginia Woolf, adapting the work of Colette, Louise Bogan, and others for the Manhattan Theatre Club, as well as curating and writing the national television series of independent films by women, *Through Her Eyes.* Sections of "The Scan Chronicles" are excerpted from her work-in-progress, *Phantom Limb,* which combines memoir and fiction. Currently she teaches in the Writing Program at the California Institute of the Arts.